# Nursing Process *in Action*

# Nursing Process *in* Action

**Pearl Gardner, EdD, RN**
Assistant Professor
The University of Texas at El Paso
College of Health Sciences, School of Nursing

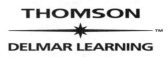

THOMSON
™
DELMAR LEARNING

Australia Canada Mexico Singapore Spain United Kingdom United States

**THOMSON**

**DELMAR LEARNING**

Nursing Process in Action
by Pearl Gardner, EdD, RN

**Executive Director,**
**Health Care Business Unit:**
William Brottmiller

**Executive Editor:**
Cathy L. Esperti

**Acquisitions Editor:**
Matthew Filimonov

**Developmental Editor:**
Marjorie A. Bruce

**Executive Marketing Manager:**
Dawn F. Gerrain

**Channel Manager:**
Jennifer McAvey

**Editorial Assistant:**
Patricia Osborn

**Production Manager:**
Barbara A. Bullock

**Art/Design Coordinator:**
Mary Colleen Liburdi

**Project Editor:**
John Mickelbank

**Production Coordinator:**
Catherine Ciardullo

Library of Congress
Cataloging-in-Publication Data

Gardner, Pearl.
  Nursing process in action / Pearl
Gardner.
    p.cm.
Includes bibliographical references and
index.
  ISBN 0-7668-2225-7
1. Nursing.   I. Title.
  RT41. G35 2002
  610.73—dc21

                              2002012236

## NOTICE TO THE READER

# DEDICATION

This text is dedicated to the beginning nursing students to whom I taught the nursing process. They inspired me with their curiosity, their questions, and their desire to learn. As they became involved with critical thinking and attempted to solve clients' problems through the use of the nursing process, they expressed the need for a book that shows how to put it all together. *Nursing Process in Action* is a result of their requests.

# Contents

# Preface

From my earliest introduction to nursing, I was excited by the nursing process—how the related parts, when carefully put together, produced a plan of care specific to a client's needs. It was then—and is now—a learned way of thinking that allows a nurse to conceptualize and implement care. A conscientious application of the nursing process hones critical thinking skills and allows a nurse to function independently in today's changing health-care environment—even one with predetermined treatment plans and managed care.

The nursing process can be complex. Indeed, in many cases it is made overly complex to the initiate, so a student misses the correlation between the component parts of the process and the desired results. This book is intended to be a clear, direct text that helps beginning students gain an understanding of the nursing process early in their careers. It has been my observation that students who readily grasp the nursing process develop into great nurses—those who develop a lifetime of good habits that serve them well in their future courses, the state board exams, and their careers.

## ORGANIZATION

This book is organized into six chapters. The first chapter provides an overview of what the nursing process is all about. It introduces the steps, shows their interrelatedness, and provides the student with an example of how the parts can be put together to formulate an individualized plan of care. This chapter also shows how critical thinking facilitates problem solving and leads to quick decision making. It introduces caring and communication as integral parts of the plan of care.

Each of the subsequent five chapters addresses one component of the nursing process. Each chapter is written to give the student a clear understanding of the significance of the specific part and its contribution to the final outcome. The latest taxonomy of the North American Nursing Diagnosis Association (NANDA) (2001–2002) is used in the text.

Chapters 2 through 6 refer to additional clinical case studies with related information and care plans. This content can be found on the Web page dedicated to *Nursing Process in Action* at **http://www.delmarhealthcare.com/nursing/olc/asp.** Examples of different approaches to assessment are introduced and care plans are subsequently developed. The pathoflow sheet is a unique feature. It is intended to create awareness of the pathophysiological, psychological, and spiritual cause and effect relationships between these components and the client's problems (nursing diagnoses). This awareness enables nurses to use a comprehensive holistic approach when providing care.

## FEATURES

Faculty and students will appreciate the following features that provide for easy readability and understanding of the content:

- The text presentation moves from the simple to the complex, allowing users to master one concept before moving to the next.
- Nursing in Action boxes are clinical situations that emphasize a main concept in the content discussion. Client scenarios, which contain critical thinking/problem solving and decision-making elements, are used in the context of the nursing process. Most chapters have Nursing in Action boxes where appropriate.
- Test Your Understanding (following Nursing in Action Case Studies where appropriate) are questions designed to enhance critical thinking skills. Answers are provided at the end of the chapter.
- Answers to Review Questions are provided in the Online Companion Web site.
- Online Companion provides additional resources that are of use to both instructors and students. The case studies (referenced in each text chapter) provide the opportunity to users to assess their understanding of text content as they develop nursing care plans. Other resources include Frequently Asked Questions (FAQs) based on text content and an instructors manual.
- Ethical/cultural/spiritual scenarios relate to discussion of these concepts within the text. They challenge the student to select the correct responses/ actions relevant to the nursing process.

# Acknowledgments

The author expresses appreciation to the following colleagues for their review comments and recommendations that contributed to the development of the text:

Netta Moncur Bowen, MS, RN. Nursing Department, Seminole Community College, Sanford, Florida

Linda R. Delunas, PhD, RN. School of Nursing, Indiana University Northwest, Gary, Indiana

Esther S. Gonzales, RN, MSN, MS Ed. Nursing Department, Del Mar College, Corpus Christi, Texas

Lynn M. Stover, DSN, RNC. Capstone College of Nursing, University of Alabama, Tuscaloosa, Alabama

ASSESSMENT

DIAGNOSIS

EVALUATION

PLANNING

IMPLEMENTATION

# The Nursing Process: A Synopsis

## OBJECTIVES

Upon completion of this chapter, you should be able to:

- Define the nursing process.
- Identify the steps of the nursing process in sequence.
- Describe the interrelatedness of each step.
- List ways in which the nursing process facilitates nursing care planning.
- Discuss critical thinking as an integral part of the nursing process.
- Describe decision making as a collaborative component of the nursing process.
- Explain how problem solving works throughout the steps of the nursing process.
- Describe attitudes of the caring nurse.
- Discuss the dangers of not putting it all together.
- Describe qualities of the caring person.
- Identify ways in which these caring behaviors can develop.
- Explain the importance of good communication in decision making.
- Explain the need for good interpersonal and intrapersonal relationships in putting the care plan together.

OBJECTIVES *continued*

- List behaviors that will control the development of an individualized care plan.
- Demonstrate understanding of the Nursing in Action case studies in:
  1. Critical thinking.
  2. Decision making.
  3. Problem solving.

## KEY TERMS

| | | |
|---|---|---|
| analyze | evaluation | intrapersonal |
| assessment | goal | intuition |
| caring | implementation | need |
| critical thinking | interpersonal | nursing process |
| diagnosis | interrelated | planning |
| empathy | intervention | prioritizing |

Students throughout their professional nursing education are required to use critical thinking, problem solving, and decision making in the delivery of patient care. Many nursing educators attempt to instill this knowledge through the teaching of the nursing process, a cyclical approach that includes assessment, diagnosis, planning, intervention, evaluation, conclusion, and reassessment. Professional nursing organizations also follow the nursing process format to test educational performance of students and graduates.

The National League for Nursing Diagnostic Tests follow this approach. These tests are designed to help students identify areas of weakness prior to completion of their nursing education. The National Council of Licensure Examination (NCLEX) is also organized according to the nursing process. For nursing students to fully grasp and apply the concepts (proposed in the nursing process), didactic and application training must begin at the very start of their educational career.

This chapter is designed to help you understand the component parts of the nursing process. It will show you how the cyclical nature of the process encourages you to critically think, problem solve, and make decisions about patient care. It focuses on the caring component of nursing and the importance of developing good psychomotor and intellectual skills in order to meet each client's needs.

Most beginning nursing students have difficulty understanding and individualizing the nursing process. This chapter should help you conceptualize the parts and their interrelatedness. The examples of actual nursing plans of care should help you understand how to put the nursing process into action, and how to put it all together.

## THE NURSING PROCESS DEFINED

What is the nursing process and what is its significance to the beginning nurse? Perhaps all of your life you wanted to become a nurse. You might have imagined yourself caring for many people and helping them to get well. Those are wonderful ideas that many nurses have but so many, when they actually begin to study nursing, find it difficult, and many do not continue. I believe this happens to many people because they have not been shown the fun of nursing and have not been helped to feel the inside joy that comes from helping people. Specific interventions and innovations can help the nursing student find joy in nursing even from the very beginning. The nursing process will help you to do this. This textbook, *Nursing Process in Action*, should not only give you in-depth understanding of the component parts of the nursing process but should help you write actual nursing plans of care, as well as implement and determine outcomes and the need for reassessment. This book is designed for easy implementation.

The nursing process is a simple model that will help you work into more complex methods. Because you will have to think critically and reason soundly, you will find yourself putting pieces together to come up with decisions about what to do to help your clients solve many problems. The nursing process will help you do this. The nursing process is a simple way of looking at the sequence of events that surround a client's **needs** and problems. You need to remember that these events can change and may even change rapidly. Hence, you must be able to identify any new developments (on a continuous basis) in order to determine if the original needs or problems have changed.

## SIGNIFICANCE OF THE NURSING PROCESS

The nursing process is client centered. That means you will need to individualize what you do for one client, that is, the one client with whom you are working at that particular time. You will need to read about things that should be done for clients with particular problems. But even if your client has the same problem, you may not be able to use this information in its solution. There may be developments in the client situation that prohibit its use. To put it succinctly, the **nursing process** is a tool that you, the nursing student, will use to systematically analyze client care data, make inferences and draw conclusions about existing problems, and determine what you can do about them. It is cyclical and sequential in that it includes assessment, which leads to diagnosing, planning, implementing, evaluating, and revision. It shows you how to stop a process when the problem is solved (goals are met), and how to rework the entire cycle when the problem is not solved (goals are not met).

The nursing process also provides you with an organized way of collecting and analyzing information about clients. It will guide you through specific and alternate ways of meeting client needs. It involves several elements that are crucial to effective nursing care. The processes of critical thinking, decision making, and problem solving help you work through the phases of the nursing process.

## PHASES OF THE NURSING PROCESS

The nursing process consists of the following phases: assessment, diagnosis, planning, prioritizing, implementation, evaluation, revision of the plan of care, and recording the plan. The nursing process is a dynamic structure that guides nursing care (Figure 1–1).

### Assessment

**Assessment** is the first part of the nursing process. It is the data collection aspect. When the client enters the health-care setting, you begin this assessment because in some way it is conveyed to you that a problem exists. You collect data from a variety of sources—client, family, chart, and health-care team (Figure 1–2). This data provides information for all the other parts of the nursing process. You will dissect this data and **analyze** it in its entirety in order to arrive at the client's problem(s). This requires in-depth thinking. You will

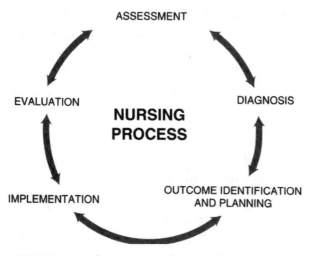

FIGURE 1–1    Components of the nursing process.

put the puzzle together and arrive at what you think is the nursing diagnosis that you then verify by standard defining characteristics. Nursing diagnoses are those problems and needs that you find by examining (critically analyzing) the assessment data. An example of a nursing diagnosis is "constipation."

## Diagnosis

The **diagnosis** is the client's problem that you identify. You give it a name selected from a list of diagnoses developed by the North American Nursing Diagnosis Association (NANDA) (see the appendix at the back of the book). Some nursing diagnoses are actual; that is, the signs and symptoms are readily

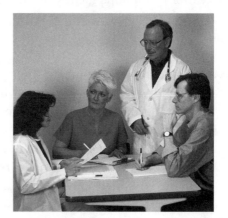

FIGURE 1–2    Nurses work collaboratively with health-care team members.

evident. Others are potential (the treatment plan may cause the patient to develop new problems). You will need to list all diagnoses in order to develop a plan to treat and a plan to prevent. Some nursing diagnoses you will be able to treat following the standard protocol. Others will require collaboration with other disciplines and your instructor.

## Planning

**Planning** consists of those things that you do to help the client now that the diagnosis has been identified. You will do this by working on these areas: **goal** setting, priority setting, identifying the nursing interventions, developing the plan of care, putting it all together, and reassessing the client before implementing the plan of care. Always reassess the client before performing the actions you choose. Continue your assessment throughout the process and record and report significant changes that might cause you not to do what you originally intended. Once you have identified the problems, you ask intuitively, "What would be appropriate for my client to accomplish?" From your answer, you formulate your goals. An example of a goal that relates to the identified diagnosis of constipation is, "The client will have a bowel movement before noon on 11/29/2002." There will be many goals. You will need to decide which one needs first attention, so you prioritize.

## Prioritizing

**Prioritizing** is putting the goals in order of urgency. You will number them one through ten (for example) and you will deal with them in this order. The tasks you perform in order to accomplish the goals are called nursing interventions. You implement your nursing interventions.

## Implementation

**Implementation** is putting the plan into action, that is, carrying out the nursing **interventions**. These are what you said you would do in order to create a change in the client's condition. Before you do this, however, you are to determine if what you planned to do is still necessary. Remember that some time will have passed since you developed your plan. It might be just several minutes but the situation might have changed within that short time. For example, you might have diagnosed "Fluid Volume Deficit" in your client. Your plan might have been to measure urinary output every hour from a Foley catheter and to give two ounces of water every hour. Between the time you developed your plan and your implementation, the physician writes an order to remove the Foley catheter. Your action would now change to "measure each voided specimen, record time of voiding and consistency of urine." You are to perform this continuous reassessment (evaluation) throughout the implementation of the plan of care. Then, at the end of your implementation phase, you are to perform your final evaluation.

These "what to do" tasks for a specific problem in order to realize your client's goal will be listed in your Nursing Care Plan Book. These are nursing skills that you should practice before implementing. Remember to seek help with these if you are uncertain.

## Evaluation

During your **evaluation** you determine if your goals are met. You critically analyze whether what you wanted to happen in this client's behalf has actually taken place (Figure 1–3). Imagine the personal satisfaction for both you and the client if it has. If it has not, don't be discouraged. Support the client, analyze your formulas, and ask why it didn't work. Begin to gather more data, use other resources, and ask your instructor or other experts for help. Probably you need to formulate a new diagnosis. Regardless of what you need to do, remember the plan is cyclical and continuous and continues to be fun, demanding, and challenging. Good luck.

## Revision of the Plan of Care

If the goals have not been met after the evaluation, then you may need to collect new data, form a new nursing diagnosis, formulate new goals, use new

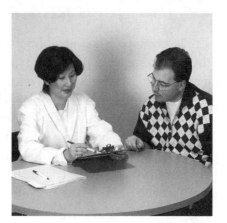

**FIGURE 1–3**   Nurse and client review outcomes.

interventions, and reevaluate. Remember that the nursing process is cyclical. Consider if things have changed since you did your first assessment. Do you have a new goal? Do you need to change your priorities? For example, you had planned to sit your client up in a chair for breakfast, as ordered by the physician. When you take the tray into the room, your client is complaining of severe pain. The pain medication that was given four hours earlier is no longer effective. You decide to give another dose of medication (according to the physician's order), and allow the client to eat in bed until the pain subsides. You make a decision to sit the client up about an hour later when he is more comfortable. Remember that assessment is continuous throughout all of your activities. You should be continuously asking if the planned goal is being realized. Do you need to do something else? An overall evaluation follows your interventions.

### Recording the Plan

Recording the plan will help you organize and will help others understand your sequencing of events. The sequencing (documentation), for example, can be done in six columns. Column one is the portion of the data that you used to support your nursing diagnosis. Column two is your nursing diagnosis, three is for goals, four for interventions, and column five is for your rationale or scientific reason for using these interventions. Column six will be saved for your evaluation. Other methods of documentation are available, and your instructor may present these to you. Record legibly so that it can be easily read and understood.

## INTERRELATEDNESS OF THE PHASES OF THE NURSING PROCESS

The **interrelatedness** shows how each phase of the nursing process builds on the preceding ones. The first part must be basically correct for all the other parts to work. This means the truth about the client's situation must be known in order to get to the real problem and to be able to deal appropriately with it. Your question should always be whether or not you are helping your client with the solution of the current problem, and whether solution of the problem is a priority for your client. Let us develop a scenario with the previous nursing diagnosis of constipation. While interviewing your client, she tells you that she has not had a "stool" in five days and that her last one was very hard. You palpate her abdomen and find it to be very firm. You think she might be constipated so you scan the NANDA list and find that constipation is included. You write in the data column, "no stool for five days, abdomen quite firm." In the diagnosis column you will write "constipation." In the goal column you will write "the client will have a bowel movement before the end of my shift," and in the intervention column you will write measures that the nurse can independently carry out to help a client have a bowel movement, such as "increase fluids." On the lunch menu you will circle foods with high fiber content.

Remember that you can only carry out these interventions if it is permissible for that client. Because you are working with a team and with your instructor, you must remember to report your findings and discuss your plan of care with these individuals. Since your client is probably quite uncomfortable, the physician will likely write an order that will help the client move her bowels quickly. You will also carry out this dependent function.

The client will very likely have a bowel movement. If she does, you will write "goal met" in the evaluation column. Remember to record the time and the consistency of the stool. Take note of how all the parts of the care plan are interrelated, from the data to the culmination with a bowel movement. (See example of completed Nursing Care Plan on page 10.)

## THE NURSING PROCESS AND FACILITATING THE NURSING CARE PLAN

The nursing process provides a way of organizing data. It also helps in data sharing among nurses and other members of the health-care team. It helps each caregiver to build on previous data instead of always starting from zero. It aids coordination and group planning through documentation and sharing. The interdisciplinary team—physician, physical therapist, occupational therapist, nutritionist, social worker—can examine a list of problems identified by the nurse and use or expand this list to provide care individually or in a collaborative manner. As you read clients' charts you are likely to see a list of nursing diagnoses written by the first nurse who examined the client. As you perform your assessment, you should determine if these problems still exist and if new problems have emerged. You may include those that you verify as current from the existing list and add the new ones you have identified as you assist the client to solve his/her problems and needs.

## Nursing Care Plan—Constipation

| Assessment | Diagnosis | Goal | Interventions | Rationale | Evaluation |
|---|---|---|---|---|---|
| Subjective: States she has not had a bowel movement (BM) for five days. Objective: Abdomen firm and tender | Constipation evidenced by: (1) No BM for five days, (2) firm and tender abdomen | Client will have a BM before 1500 today April 4. | **Independent** Give 100 cc of water every hour (not NPO) and ambulate as ordered; assist to select foods high in fiber. **Collaborative** If no BM in 4 hours, discuss possibility of getting an order from the doctor for an enema. **Dependent** Administered enema as ordered. | (1) Water softens stool and provides for easier passage of bowel contents. (2) Ambulation (activity) increases peristalsis and abdominal muscle tone. This helps the bowel to empty its contents of stool. (3) High fiber foods with sufficient water adds bulk and softness to stool and facilitates defecation. (4) An enema increases bowel contents causing irritation and evacuation of stool. | Goal met. Client had a large formed brown stool. Expressed satisfaction with the procedure. |

## CRITICAL THINKING AND THE NURSING PROCESS

Critical thinking is an integral part of the nursing process. Alfaro-LeFevre (1995) describes critical thinking as goal directed and purposeful. Allan (1997) is in concert with this idea and further defines critical thinking as a process that is not visible but engages the mental activity of the nurse and other members of the interdisciplinary team in all of their interactions with the client and the family.

In these contexts you are intuitively asking specific questions and seeking definite answers about the client care situation. Critical thinking involves clinical reasoning and the use of moral and ethical judgments (Figure 1–4). These will guide you into drawing conclusions about needed nursing interventions in given client care situations. Critical thinking also encourages analysis and differentiation of facts as opposed to that which is fictitious, unreliable, and nonrelevant client data, and should result in sound decision making about client outcomes.

According to Miller and Babcock (1996), **critical thinking** is "viewing situations from different perspectives to develop an in-depth, comprehensive understanding." So you are going to think deeply and questioningly. You are going to examine new and previous developments to determine whether you will work with what you identified as the original problem or whether you

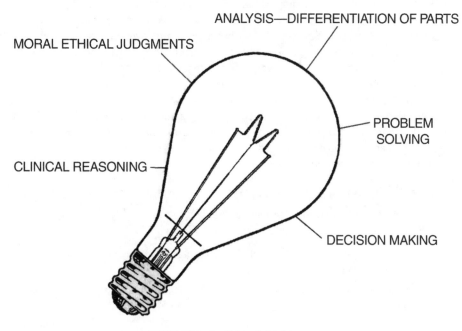

FIGURE 1–4   Critical thinking.

should now think through a new problem. A first requirement of nursing is to learn to relax and enjoy thinking. Think analytically, critically, creatively, and effectively. These parameters of critical thinking should help you to arrive at favorable conclusions about your client's problems and/or needs, and should guide you to find effective solutions. You will find these solutions through reading and from asking questions of your instructors and the medical and nursing team (see the following Critical Thinking Case Study).

## Critical Thinking Case Study

You are assigned to care for Mrs. Bryant, a 45-year-old female client. At 0730 you checked her vital signs. They were all in normal range. She answered your questions appropriately and was oriented to time, place, and person. Her color was pink, she denied pain, and you saw no obvious sign of distress. She elected to do her own morning care. As you leave the room, you tell her you will bring her breakfast at 0800. Dr. Barnes enters as you are leaving. You return to the room at the stated time carrying her tray with everything that she ordered for breakfast. You find Mrs. Bryant with her head buried in her hands as she sobs loudly. You begin to think that she might have received bad news from home because her telephone is on her bed. You place the tray on her bedside stand, but she screams, "I do not want to eat, I am not hungry!" Instead of discussing her food choices you place a firm hand on her right shoulder. You remain quiet and allow her to cry (empathy/ understanding). You collect data, remembering that Dr. Barnes had just left her room and that you had not heard her telephone ring. You wonder if she made a call. After fifteen minutes she stops sobbing. She is now quiet and you are thinking critically. You wonder what Dr. Barnes told her. She realizes that you care because you have spent the last fifteen minutes in silent support, developing a relationship of trust. You ask Mrs. Bryant if Dr. Barnes gave her any information. She replies, "Yes, he told me that I have cancer." You now begin to explore measures that will assist Mrs. Bryant to cope throughout the treatment process of a long-term illness.

### TEST YOUR UNDERSTANDING

Read the Critical Thinking Case Study and respond to the statements, **T** for true and **F** for false.

1. Dr. Barnes should have been called back to the client's room to support her until she calmed down.

2. Mrs. Bryant probably wanted to call a family member but was too overwhelmed to do so.

*continues*

---

**Critical Thinking Case Study** *continued*

3. The crying probably relieved some of Mrs. Bryant's stress.

4. Fifteen minutes is a long time to stay with a client.

5. The charge nurse should have been called immediately to explain the diagnosis to Mrs. Bryant.

6. You should have removed Mrs. Bryant's tray and recorded on her chart, "refused to eat, not hungry."

7. When Mrs. Bryant begins to eat, she should be encouraged to eat the total complement of her breakfast.

8. You should suggest that Mrs. Bryant call another physician to get a second opinion.

9. You should call Mrs. Bryant's husband and ask him to come to be with his wife immediately.

10. You should ask Mrs. Bryant if she had cancer before.

The correct answers can be found on page 39.

## DECISION MAKING: A COLLABORATIVE COMPONENT OF THE NURSING PROCESS

A major component of the nursing process is decision making. Through critical thinking you mentally process information. Now you must make decisions about the actions that are needed, permissible, and correct for your client. The American Nurses Association and the Canadian Nurses Association set the standards that guide the nurse into acceptable and safe practice. According to Alfaro-LeFevre (1998), these standards are written for specialty areas, such as the Association of Critical Care Nurses and the Association of Operating Room Nurses. Agencies often write their own standards. You should study these carefully and follow the guidelines after you make your decisions and before you carry out your nursing actions. You must remember that some decisions require immediate action, whereas other interventions can be done later. This is called priority setting. It involves continuous assessment and may require collaboration with your instructor. You need to be adaptable and have the ability to manipulate equipment in order to perform nursing skills. This comes through practice. Remember to use problem solving when making your decisions.

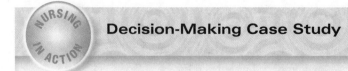

## Decision-Making Case Study

Mr. John Jones, a 24-year-old client, had an appendectomy and exploratory laparotomy for a ruptured appendix. You are caring for Mr. Jones on his first postoperative day. You review his orders that read: (1) remove Foley catheter in A.M., (2) ambulate client in room, (3) offer full liquid diet. As you perform your morning assessment of Mr. Jones, you notice that: (1) his urine is bloody, and (2) he vomited the water he had requested fifteen minutes earlier. Although you had thoroughly reviewed the procedure for Foley catheter removal in the hospital procedure book, you would refrain from removing the catheter because there are now new developments since the physician wrote the order for removal. You would not ambulate Mr. Jones because he is probably bleeding, and you had previously read in your nursing text that one intervention for bleeding was bed rest. You also replaced his tray with the full liquids on the breakfast cart because you read in your nursing text that an independent function (which the nurse can initiate) is nothing by mouth (NPO) when a client is vomiting. You have now made three wise decisions based on scientific facts. Your next step is to report your findings to your instructor and to the professional staff. You should now wait for new orders. You will perform similar assessment and evaluation before carrying out the new orders.

### TEST YOUR UNDERSTANDING

Read the Decision-Making Case Study and respond to the statements, **T** for true, **F** for false, and **NA** for those that are not applicable.

1. While caring for Mr. Jones it is important for the nurse to recognize that he had surgery the day before.

2. The nurse should read all postoperative orders written by the physician before beginning to care for Mr. Jones.

3. The Foley catheter should be removed because it is the physician's order.

4. The bloody urine was due to acute nephritis.

5. There was no need to measure the urine since it was bloody.

6. Mr. Jones would develop complications if he were not ambulated that day as ordered.

7. The vomiting was probably due to the anesthesia he received while in the operating room and was of no significance on his first day after surgery.

8. Mr. Jones can be expected to stop vomiting that morning.

9. If Mr. Jones complains of thirst after the vomiting, he should be given orange juice.

10. Mr. Jones' height and weight should be taken before he is fed.

The correct answers can be found on page 39.

## PROBLEM SOLVING IN THE NURSING PROCESS

All the parts of the nursing process are geared to assisting clients to solve problems. If you stop to reflect, you will realize that you have solved major and minor problems in your own life. In the profession of nursing you assist clients in solving their problems. This will give great satisfaction to both you and your clients. One advantage that you may have in helping clients solve problems is that professional standards, guidelines, and protocol are set for you. You should have fun as you put cognitive, affective, and psychomotor behaviors (or skills) into practice. You should have a good feeling. You will see the health of your clients improve and you may even feel the great satisfaction that professional nurses feel. Now look at Table 1–1 to see how the nursing process and problem solving work hand in hand.

### TABLE 1–1

**Comparison of the Nursing Process and Problem-Solving Approaches**

| Nursing Process | Problem-Solving |
|---|---|
| • Assessment is using all available data to draw conclusions about a problem. | • Look at all available data with the intent of finding the problem. |
| • Diagnosis is selecting the problem and categorizing it by name. | • Examine the data and find the problem. |
| • Planning is deciding how to solve the problem. | • Draw conclusions about the approach to be used to solve the problem. |
| • Implementation is carrying out the developed plan. | |
| • Evaluation is determining if the plan was successful in achieving the desired outcome. | • Use the planned approach. |
| | • Decide if the problem is resolved and if further work is necessary. |

### Problem-Solving Case Study

You are assigned to care for Mrs. Janice Black, a 55-year-old female who was admitted with a diagnosis of chronic foot ulcer. During your early morning assessment you notice that tears are running down Mrs. Black's cheeks. You ask her

*continues*

## Problem-Solving Case Study *continued*

if she is in pain. She says, "Yes, I am hurting very badly." On further questioning she identifies the location of the pain at the site of the ulcer, the severity as nine on a scale of one to ten (with ten being most severe), and the nature of the pain as throbbing and burning. You remember that when you read your nursing process data on pain assessment it said the client in pain might complain of pain and might also demonstrate pain behaviors such as grimacing and restlessness. To the contrary, Mrs. Black is motionless and by this time her gown is wet with perspiration as her tears flow freely and continuously. You begin to problem solve. You conclude that if Mrs. Black has pain at this moment, it is not her most pressing concern. You sit beside her bed, hold her hand, gently wipe her tears, and ask permission to change her gown. She agrees. You ask if she would like to talk with you about another problem other than her pain. She agrees. You draw the curtains to secure privacy. You lean forward and hold Mrs. Black's hand. You ask, "Is there something you want to tell me?" She replies, "Yes, I have no money to pay my rent and I am going to be evicted from my apartment." You have used the problem-solving technique to arrive at the client's priority problem. You will now use the decision-making process to decide on the agencies that can help Mrs. Black and the techniques necessary to get the right people involved.

### TEST YOUR UNDERSTANDING

Read the Problem-Solving Case Study and respond to the statements, **T** for true and **F** for False.

1. The nurse should have given Mrs. Black the pain medication without further investigation.
2. The pain remained Mrs. Black's first priority.
3. Mrs. Black probably had pain, but this took second priority.
4. The pain problem should have been addressed after the first priority problem.
5. Mrs. Black disclosed her inner feelings after a trust relationship developed between her and the student.
6. The student's behavior demonstrated caring.
7. Holding Mrs. Black's hand demonstrated empathy.
8. The nurse should assist Mrs. Black to explore her resources for solving her problem.
9. Family members could be one resource for Mrs. Black.
10. Mrs. Black should be helped to explore long-term solutions to her problem.

The answers can be found on page 39.

**Nursing Process Case Study**

**Integrating Critical Thinking, Decision Making, and Problem Solving**
You (the nursing student) are assigned to Mr. Ray, a 54-year-old client on
4 North/East. At 0730, you find him lying in semi-Fowler's position. His face is
flushed and his breathing is rapid at 38 per minute. The nasal cannula for his
oxygen is hanging below his chin. You approach him, calling his name. You say,
"Good Morning, Mr. Ray." He attempts to answer in a groan. Because he is very
short of breath, you ask, "May I adjust your oxygen for you?" You attempt to lift
the cannula but you quickly drop it when he shouts, "Leave it alone!" He gets
more agitated by the minute. The nurse's aide walks in with his breakfast tray. He
looks at it cross-eyed and closes his eyes. As she leaves the room she mutters,
"miserable and uncooperative." You are saddened by Mr. Ray's behavior but
become deeply concerned as you watch his breathing become more difficult.
Intuitively, you gaze at him from the foot of his bed. You begin to think. He came
in with a diagnosis of chronic obstructive pulmonary disease (COPD) of eight
years' duration (information from chart). If he had not wanted treatment, he would
not have agreed to hospitalization. Then you ask, "Mr. Ray, is there anything I can
do for you?" (critical thinking). Almost gasping, he replies, "Find my keys. I don't
know who has them. My apartment is open." You now begin the process of
problem solving. You remember that in the morning report the night nurse had
said he was brought in by ambulance. As you leave the room, Mr. Ray allows your
partner, another nursing student, to put his oxygen in place. Now he has developed a trust relationship. He believes you will come back with his keys. You
quickly review the medical records and find that he lives alone. He had managed
to call 911 Emergency Service from his cellular phone. White Acres Ambulance
Service brought him to the hospital. You make the decision to call White Acres
Ambulance Service and ask about the keys. The driver tells you that Mr. Ray might
have been too sick to remember giving him the keys and asking him to lock his
door. The driver stated that he would bring the keys to the hospital in approximately
twenty minutes.

As you relay the incident to your instructor and the team leader, a messenger
puts the keys in your hand. Expectantly, you walk into Mr. Ray's room. Lifting
his hand, you put the keys in his palm. He smiles through a quick gasp, as a
tear runs down his cheek. He relaxes and says, "Please tighten my catheter
and please give me my breakfast." He then whispers, "Do you want to take
my temperature?" As you say, "Yes, thank you," you reflect on the positive
outcome of your critical-thinking, problem-solving, and decision-making
approach. With better understanding and **empathy** you care for Mr. Ray the
rest of the day.

Your actions represented the nursing process in action:

1. You collected data from various sources (the client, the chart, the ambulance driver).
2. You arrived at a nursing diagnosis of: "High anxiety state related to client's lost keys, evidenced by agitation, increased respiration, and refusal to eat."
3. You developed your goal: Client's anxiety will be mild to moderate within 45 minutes or less after his keys are found.
4. You planned your strategy to find the keys.
5. You implemented your strategy.
6. You evaluated your goals and wrote, "goals met," evidenced by client's calm demeanor almost immediately after he was given his keys. You shared at post conference and anxiously waited to return to clinical the next day because you "loved it." Hear yourself saying, "Nursing is for me. I have chosen the right profession."

## Problem Solving Using Trial and Error and Intuition

Sometimes the professional staff will use trial and error and intuition to solve problems. It is good to become familiar with these approaches, but remember you are too inexperienced to use them at this time.

### Trial and Error

With the trial-and-error approach the nurse tries many ways to solve the problem. Because these ways are not scientifically proven, they may or may not work. Many times they are not time expedient and may even be detrimental to the client. Practice based on scientific evidence and standards is always best.

### Intuition

**Intuition** is an inner feeling that nurses develop. It tells them that something is wrong or is about to happen. Nurses should not ignore their intuition but should act on it promptly. By so doing they may prevent complications and may even save clients' lives. If you, as a beginning student, have an intuitive feeling, do not ignore it. Tell your instructor, who will help you explore your thoughts and the situation further. Often, intuition results from unconscious assessment and data analysis based on experience.

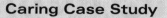

### Intuition Case Study

I would like to relate an experience of a beginning student to you. It was about midmorning on a clinical day when a student and I stood in a quiet corner of the hospital unit discussing her client care plans. Suddenly the student said, "I must go." She ran into her client's room; I followed. On quick observation we found no obvious change in the client's condition. He was eating lunch. Minutes later the patient began to cough. There was sudden vomiting and his face and chest became covered with blood. The medical and nursing team raced to the client's room at the student's call. We quickly transferred Mr. Reed to the intensive care unit where he was placed on a respirator. An MRI (magnetic resonance imaging) revealed a tear in his esophagus that occurred when he vomited. Remember, even beginning students can have intuitive feelings. When you have one, don't ignore it.

## THE NURSING PROCESS: A CARING PARADIGM

As you develop an understanding of the nursing process, you will have one basic question in mind; that is, what can I do to help? You will be very careful about what you say and how to say what you want to say. You will view your client with empathy. This means you will develop an in-depth understanding of the client's feelings and concerns and demonstrate the ability to share understanding through verbal and nonverbal communication and skill performance. You will find yourself searching for ways to improve your client's condition. These internal feelings are called caring. Watson and Ray (1988) describe the process of nursing as human caring, while Leininger (1995) states that "caring is essential to curing and pervades all efforts to help an individual recover after an illness and be cured."

### Caring Case Study

The beginning nursing student walked into his client's room. There he found a woman, cold and clammy, with a temperature of 95°F. She had a Foley catheter in place with concentrated urine of 25 cc per hour, and an IV of 5 percent dextrose in

*continues*

**Caring Case Study** *continued*

water. The client's lips were cracked and her skin was dry and scaling. The nursing student had read the client's chart and saw that she had pneumonia. She had already been in the hospital for nine (9) days. In the morning report, the student had heard that the client refused to eat for the past two days and had not had a bowel movement for five days. When he realized that the client was only 63 years old, the student said to his instructor, "I am doing something about this today." He formulated the following nursing diagnoses:

- Fluid Volume Deficit—evidenced by concentrated urine, cracked lips, and dry skin.
- Nutrition—less than body requirements related to poor intake of food.
- Elimination Altered—evidenced by concentrated urinary output, of 50 cc in two hours, and no bowel movement for five days.

Since the client was coherent, the nursing student asked her what her goals were for the day. She gave no reply, but he shared his goals for her. He informed the client that the goals could only be accomplished if they worked on them together. Before the shift was over, the client's intake was 120 cc of pineapple juice and 400 cc of orange juice (fluids of her choice). She had eaten the fruit from her dinner tray and agreed to be propped up at a 45-degree angle instead of 30. The client was deep breathing and her urinary output was approximately 30 cc per hour. The student began to shout, "All goals met." The student's face flushed with excitement that seemed to demonstrate true human caring. The charge nurse admitted that the client's condition had definitely improved. So you see, the beginning nursing student can make an impact through caring.

## Developing Attitudes of Caring

**Caring** is a feeling of wanting to help. It is a propelling force that tells us that something needs to be done. It identifies the urgency of a situation and propels us to action. It is conveyed through expressions and actions. It conveys determination and empathy to the receiver. This in turn creates trust in the client, which emerges into a trusting relationship between the caregiver and the client.

According to Leininger (1995), "caring is the most important and central focus of nursing." It encompasses "those human acts and processes which provide assistance to another individual or group based on an interest in, or concern for, that human being." In this context, as the nursing student you will develop a cognitive awareness of patients' problems and needs. You will formulate outcome goals and objectives, and intervene appropriately to support, alleviate, and meet identified needs. Watson and Ray (1988) advocate that we first love and care for ourselves, so as a beginning nurse you are to believe in yourself, identify your strengths, and put your abilities to work. A study of Watson's "Ten Caring Factors" should help you develop the attributes of a caring nurse.

**Watson's Ten Caring Factors**

1. Forming and acting from a humanistic/altruistic system of values.
2. Enabling and sustaining faith/hope.
3. Sensitivity to self and others.
4. Developing helping, trusting, caring relationships.
5. Promoting and accepting the expression of positive and negative feelings and emotions.
6. Engaging in a creative, individualized problem-solving, caring process.
7. Promoting transpersonal teaching/learning.
8. Attending to supportive, protective and/or corrective mental, physical, social, and spiritual environment.
9. Assisting with the gratification of basic human needs while preserving human dignity and wholeness.
10. Allowing for and being open to existential, phenomenological, and spiritual dimensions of caring and healing that cannot be explained scientifically.

As you put these into practice you should feel the satisfaction that comes from caring.

## Qualities of the Caring Nurse

Caring qualities can never be hidden. They are evident in every encounter with a client and enhance client care outcomes. That is, most clients demonstrate less anxiety, are more compliant to therapy, and enter into a health-care contract more readily in an atmosphere of caring. Some of the qualities of the caring nurse are:

- Calmness under stress—does not convey an attitude of undue haste.
- Mild to moderate anxiety even in difficult situations.
- Empathy understanding or the giving of oneself demonstrated by warmth.
- Listening attentively and giving your full attention during the communication process.
- Answering questions promptly and truthfully.

- Performing only those skills with which you are comfortable and competent.
- Maintaining patient confidentiality by sharing information only with the medical and nursing team.
- Paying attention to details that include client's and family's comfort and a clean and attractive environment.
- Answering questions from a sound scientific base.
- Observing privacy when necessary.
- Believing in yourself.
- Displaying confidence.
- Making only contracts that are relevant to the client's well-being.
- Keeping promises. For example, returning to the client's room at the time promised.

## Developing Behaviors that Demonstrate Caring

The fact that you have chosen to be a nurse says that you have that inner motivation to share, to give, and to care. At this point of your career your sharing potential might be limited, but the purpose of your nursing education is to provide you with the knowledge and skills that will broaden this potential. Let us look at the content areas to which you will be exposed and determine how they will enhance your caring ability:

- **Anatomy and Physiology**—Helps you to understand structures, organs, and functions of the body, so you can understand health alterations, correctly name necessary ones for your client, and communicate more effectively with all who are involved in client care.
- **Pathophysiology**—Gives you information on the processes within the body that result in signs and symptoms your client may be experiencing. By this you will inform the client whether the condition is improving or worsening and what further measures need to be followed. You will be better prepared to observe your client's condition and intervene early if changes occur.
- **Microbiology and Chemistry**—Helps you to interpret laboratory data and collaborate in the choice of antibiotics and dietary plans.
- **Pharmacology**—Provides information on drug therapy, its effectiveness and side effects, and enables client teaching on an individual basis. Improves observational skills and enables prompt intervention if evidence of side effects appears.

- **Health Promotion**—Gives you insight into the broad fields of nursing responsibilities, not only when the person is sick, but that caring extends also to the person without a medical diagnosis. For example, caring can be demonstrated in the teaching of self-breast examination. Promoting wellness is caring of a high order.
- **Growth and Development**—Provides information on the nursing needs of clients of all age groups (age continuum). It helps to differentiate the caring approach necessary for the various clients to achieve greater success with interventions.
- **Culture and Ethics**—People of different cultures and ethical beliefs may behave differently and have different expectations. You will need to study these variations in order to show respect in your caring activities. Respect can open lines of communication with clients.
- **Communication**—You will learn that communication is basic to nursing and how to use therapeutic communication in nursing care.
- **Mental Health**—In this context people are presented as psychosocial beings and you will be taught how to care using a holistic approach.
- **Teaching and Learning**—You will be exposed to the principles of teaching and learning and made to understand that every nurse is a teacher. This is the role you will play in every teaching/learning situation.
- **Research**—You will learn to determine ways in which new research findings enhance client care.
- **Technology**—Varied technological approaches will demonstrate advances in health care and you will better appreciate the benefits of good client care.
- **Group Dynamics**—The delivery of nursing is a team effort. Through exposure to group dynamics you will learn both the singular and collaborative role of every team member. You will learn to value the contributions of each team member. Mutual respect among team members is translated into security for the client, easing anxiety.
- **Problem Solving and Critical Thinking**—Exercises in analytical thought and problem identification will help you unravel client situations.
- **Diagnostic Testing**—You will study procedures and test results and be able to give correct information to clients regarding their illness.
- **Nursing Diagnosis and Nursing Process**—You will be taught how to use the cyclical approach to identify client problems and how to solve them effectively.
- **Disease Process**—Discussion of disease causation, prognosis, progression, and cure will provide you with a perspective of nursing responsibilities and client needs.

- **Nursing Care**—The study of nursing care will give you a broad perspective of the world of nursing, the contributions nurses make in the health-care arena, and the skills and motivation to provide quality care.
- **Skills and Performance**—There are many and varied skills that require nursing competence. These you will learn through discussion and hands-on practice. You will need to develop expertise in the manipulation of equipment in order to give quality care.

## IMPORTANCE OF GOOD COMMUNICATION IN DECISION MAKING

Communication is the exchange of ideas between two or more people (Kozier et al., 2000). Good communication refers to information that is factual, reliable, and open. Open communication and free exchange of ideas and issues form the basis for correct client care decisions. Because of the multifaceted nature of the health-care setting, client information is shared among many people, and various methods are used to convey messages. All of these messages culminate in decisions about the client.

As a student you will need to read carefully, understand clearly, and write legibly. Others will depend on the information that you convey to make decisions about the client. You will need to be sure that the message sent to you by a health-care messenger is the correct message and the message that was intended. You will need to repeatedly clarify information by asking questions and rereading written orders. Remember to ask for help from experts when information is unclear. The nursing process requires good communication from one component to the next so that the right client care decisions can be made.

### Poor Communication Case Study

The student nurse to whom Mr. Upton, a 55-year-old client, was assigned was in his room measuring vital signs. The patient had had a prostatectomy the day before. Mr. Upton's physician came to the room and told the student to discontinue everything and ambulate the client. The student discontinued the intravenous infusion, the continuous bladder irrigation, and the Foley catheter.

*continues*

**Poor Communication Case Study** *continued*

The physician then stopped at the desk and told the RN the same thing. Because of her years of experience, she knew that the Foley catheter should not be removed on the first postoperative day because the client could form clots and could even hemorrhage. When the RN reported this concern to the physician who had already left the unit, he admitted giving the student that information but said he did not want the catheter removed. He returned to the unit and replaced the catheter. It is important that you clarify all communication before making client care decisions. Remember to have physicians write all orders before carrying out procedures.

## Importance of Interpersonal and Intrapersonal Relationships in Putting the Care Plan Together

According to Lindberg and others (1994), **intrapersonal** communication involves interpretation of messages within the individual, whereas **interpersonal** communication occurs between two or more people. Both types of communication are important in nursing, because nurses need to examine their feelings about specific nursing issues and resolve any personal bias before they can be free to make a commitment to clients. The nurse also needs to develop good interpersonal skills, so that there is easy interaction in a stress-reduced environment. When these parameters are operating, people work together to gather client data, identify problems, write client-centered goals, and select appropriate nursing interventions. Together they await outcomes and critically analyze results.

As a nursing student you are to examine your prejudices and deal with them honestly. As you do self-examination and study cultural variations, you will be able to gain better understanding of people's unique behaviors. You will honestly collect data on different peoples and document them honestly, and through the study of cultural diversity you will formulate a plan of care that is specific and individualized to each client in your care. You will also need to address spiritual needs and provide care that is ethically sound.

### Cultural Considerations

In developing your care plan you will need to be sensitive to client's needs that are dictated by cultural orientation. This will help you assist in the resolution of their problems with greater client participation and satisfaction. This should also result in your interventions being more efficient and timely.

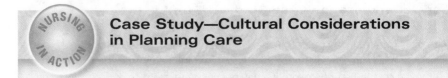

### Case Study—Cultural Considerations in Planning Care

Mr. Henry Ruiz is a 60-year-old client who has had type II diabetes for five years. He controlled this condition with oral hypoglycemics until two weeks ago when he developed pneumonia. He was admitted with a diagnosis of viral pneumonia and hyperglycemia. His blood sugar on admission was 410. He is ordered an 1800-calorie diabetic diet (ADA), 40 units of NPH insulin daily, and a sliding scale of regular insulin according to blood sugar level. He eats only about 25 percent of each meal stating that he cannot eat the hospital food "because he is not accustomed to eating that way." He had an insulin reaction on the second night of his hospitalization.

### PLAN OF CARE FOR MR. RUIZ (Cultural Considerations)

**Assessment Data**
Subjective: "I cannot eat that food. I am not used to eating that way."
Objective:

* Blood sugar 410 on admission.
* Eats only about 25 percent of each meal.
* Insulin reaction on second night of admission.

**Diagnosis Nutrition**
* Less than body requirement related to inadequate food intake evidenced by insulin reaction

**Goal**
Mr. R. will:
* Identify food idiosyncrasies.
* Identify foods that he likes to eat and will eat.
* Identify food restrictions on a diabetic diet.

**Interventions**
Ask Mr. Ruiz to name foods he does not like and to which he is allergic.
* Identify his favorite foods.
* Identify food that should be avoided on a diabetic diet.
* List food he generally eats over a 24-hour period, including breakfast, lunch, supper, and all snacks.
* Report findings to dietician.
* Ask dietician to visit Mr. Ruiz.
* Report findings and collaborate all subsequent meals and provide supplements.
* Explain insulin administration in relationship to dietary intake.

*continues*

## Case Study—Cultural Considerations *continued*

### Evaluation
* Goals met. Mr. Ruiz states that he does not like lettuce, tomatoes, baked potatoes, and meat loaf. He likes "most kinds of beans but prefers pintos." He likes squash, spinach, cucumbers, and green onions.
* Accepted the diet planned with the dietician; now eats 90 to 95 percent of all meals.
* Voiced understanding of the relationship between insulin and diet in the control of diabetes.

## Ethical Considerations

As you plan care you should be aware of ethical issues and deal with these to the satisfaction and benefit of your client. The ANA Standards of Professional Performance stresses the right of patients to collaborate with health-care givers in their plan of care and the right to make decisions (see Chapter 4).

### Case Study—Ethical Decision Making in Planning Care

Mrs. Eugenie Walters, a 36-year-old client, has multiple sclerosis. She fell and fractured her left hip. The client had no knowledge of this but she was constantly complaining of left hip pain. A month after the fall she was admitted to the hospital for extreme depression and confusion. She continued to complain about the pain while in the hospital. An X ray of the left hip revealed dislocation. The doctor discussed an open reduction and internal fixation of the hip with the client and her husband. She was favorable to the decision and signed the consent forms. On the morning of the surgery you are Mrs. Walters' student nurse. On attempting to give her a bath she says, "You may do whatever you want to do but I am not going to surgery today." She is grasping her left hip as if in pain. Her facial expression shows sadness.

#### PLAN OF CARE FOR MRS. WALTERS (Ethical Decision Making)

#### Assessment Data
Subjective: "I am not going to surgery today."
Objective: Grasping left hip: sad facial expression

*continues*

---

**Case Study - Ethical Decision Making in Planning Care** *continued*

---

**Nursing Diagnosis**
Noncompliant with medical regimen

**Goal**
Client will verbalize her concerns about the surgery.

**Interventions**
- Complete the client's bath while encouraging her to voice her feelings.
- Do not attempt to convince her to have the surgery.
- Report the development to your instructor and the charge nurse.

**Evaluation**
As client verbalized she said she wanted to wait several days before the surgery.

## Meeting Spiritual Needs

Remember that many clients have problems that relate to physical well-being, emotional state, social concerns, and spiritual needs. All of these areas must be addressed in the plan of care.

**Case Study—Meeting Spiritual Needs**

Mrs. Martinez, a 58-year-old client, is diagnosed with cancer of the rectum. She is scheduled for surgery (abdominal peritoneal resection of the rectum with a colostomy). You are the student caring for her. While taking her vital signs, you tell her that her surgery is scheduled for 10:00 A.M. and that you are there to answer her questions and to assist her to get ready. She replies by saying: "I am not afraid, I have complete confidence in God that He will see me through this ordeal. If it is my time to go, I am resigned to this. He knows best. Will you please pray for me?" Client is relaxed and demonstrates no agitation.

PLAN OF CARE FOR MRS. MARTINEZ (Meeting Spiritual Needs)

**Assessment Data**
Subjective:
Client states: "I am not afraid. I have complete confidence in God. If it is my time, He knows best. Please pray for me."

*continues*

---

**Case Study - Meeting Spiritual Needs** *continued*

Objective: Relaxed; demonstrating no agitation

**Nursing Diagnosis**
(1) Coping, effective (meeting spiritual needs effectively)
(2) Hopefulness (meeting spiritual needs effectively)

**Goal**
- Client will continue to express confidence in her spiritual belief.
- She will continue to express hopefulness in God.
- Will continue to demonstrate calm, relaxed demeanor.

**Interventions**
- Use effective communication techniques to help client to verbalize her inner feelings, empathy, listening, restatement acceptance.
- Pray with client or read from client's prayer book, Gideon's Bible, or invite the chaplain to pray.

**Evaluation**
- Client still calm on leaving unit at 0940 (accompanied by student nurse). Repeatedly said, "thank you."

See the completed care plan, including physical, ethical, cultural, and spiritual considerations in the appendix on Delmar's Web site.

---

## Dangers of Not Putting It All Together

All aspects of the nursing process are interdependent. Incomplete data can cause the formulation of an incorrect nursing diagnosis. For example, you may conclude that a client's nursing diagnosis is altered nutrition: more than body requirements. If you collect data only about the client's height and weight and fail to get information about his ideal body weight, the wrong diagnosis will lead to inappropriate planning (goals). For example, you may ask the client to identify foods and activities that will enhance weight loss. You may have the client eat two meals a day and negotiate with the dietician for a low-carbohydrate, high-protein diet. The evaluation may show that goals are met but this could be to the detriment of the client's health. Anemia, inappropriate weight loss, and a depressed immune system may result. The high-protein diet may be damaging to the client's kidneys. Inappropriate goals will lead to bad interventions.

The scenario presented above is very grave although it related to only one sample of incomplete data. To avoid critical and legal problems, collect complete data from a wide variety of sources—family members, nurses, physicians, and interdisciplinary team members—and verify from your textbook (scientific data). Always assess and reassess before beginning to process information for patient care.

## BEHAVIORS THAT CONTROL THE DEVELOPMENT OF AN INDIVIDUALIZED PLAN OF CARE

The nursing process with its component parts is intended to give the student the general information needed to: (1) collect data, (2) identify problems, (3) formulate client goals, (4) select interventions, and (5) evaluate the goals. You need to remember that these are truly guidelines. They cannot be automatically used for your clients. Each client is an individual and is unique, hence, the reason for critical thinking. You must ask, does this information that I am reading in this text relate precisely to my client? How is my client's situation different from the material I am reading? The information that you gather (using the instructions from your nursing process book) must be individualized to your client. The examples of written goals may be unrealistic for your client and the interventions may not be applicable. Your client data is likely to be different. The only section of the nursing process book that can likely be used as it is written is the rationale (the scientific reason for your action). Your client can only benefit as you develop the plan of care specifically to meet the needs of the individual you are working with at that particular time.

For example, in your nursing process book you read a nursing diagnosis of "Risk for altered respiratory function." The goals are listed as:

- Perform hourly deep-breathing exercises and cough sessions as needed.
- Demonstrate satisfactory respiratory function (tidal volume, vital capacity, forced end-expiratory volume).
- Relate importance of daily pulmonary exercises. (Carpenito, 1995, p. 747).

Assume that it is correct to select this nursing diagnosis for your client because of immobility. It is correct to arbitrarily choose the goals: (1) perform hourly deep-breathing exercises and (2) relate importance of daily pulmonary exercises. You could not, however, include the goal "cough sessions as needed" if your client, though immobile, had a complicating condition where coughing was restricted (such as surgical conditions involving the palate). Additionally, you could not include "adequate tidal volume, vital capacity, and forced end-expiratory volume," unless the specific pulmonary function tests that measure these volumes were ordered for the client. This would be unlikely. So in your use of the goal, "demonstrates satisfactory pulmonary function," you should show how these would be measured. You could say, "demonstrates satisfactory pulmonary function, evidenced by pink color, normal respiratory rate (16–20), skin warm and dry, no shortness of breath on exertion, absence of crackles and rales on auscultation." You had to use discrimination in selecting the goals from the care plan book because of the individual differences in your client's health history. Begin by deciding how your client's case differs from the written instructions. Remember that these have a more general application. You need to be specific and to individualize.

## Evaluation of Student Care Plans

Review the scenario in order to understand how grading of care plans by instructors is often based on how well the plan is individualized for a specific patient.

A true incident: Sarah Hamilton (not the real name), a beginning nursing student, received a grade of 80 percent for her care plan. Her friend Linda Parker received a grade of 65. Linda accused the instructor of bias and prejudice. She complained that she had done the care plan exactly like Sarah's but the instructor had elected to give her a failing grade. The instructor was aware of the difference in the clients' diagnoses. Both clients were overweight by more than fifty pounds. The nursing diagnosis for both clients was correctly identified as altered nutrition: more than body requirement, evidenced by an excess of fifty pounds. Sarah's client was ordered a regular diet after surgery to remove prostheses of the right knee. She would have further surgery after approximately three months. During this time she was to be treated with antibiotics and encouraged to lose weight while at home. Sarah's short-term goal for this particular nursing diagnosis was that the client would discuss the importance of losing weight. Her long-term goal read, "client will plan a diet that is low in calories and high in protein, fiber, and fluids." Her interventions involved a dietary recall and identifying food idiosyncrasies of her patient. Linda had the identical information in her care plan but her client had a total gastrectomy for cancer of the stomach and was NPO. The individualized care plan is written prior to caring for a client. It is generally planned the night before and implemented the next day. It is obvious Linda did not understand the nursing process or the meaning of "individualize." It is also apparent that she failed to effectively care for her client. She was told that she should have received zero for her care plan. Her peers agreed.

Thus, all nursing actions and behaviors should focus on the individual client's assessment.

- Assessment should focus on physical examination, interview, and data collected from the client's record.
- The nursing diagnosis should be formulated from what the client says during the interview (subjective data) and what is found during the physical examination (objective data). The nursing diagnosis should be named from the NANDA list as it applies to the client. Defining characteristics that you will find in your nursing process book should substantiate this. At least three matching characteristics with your subjective and/or objective data are required for your nursing diagnosis to be correct.

The goals (what you would like your client to accomplish) should be individualized and attainable by that person. The interventions should be those that can be implemented by and for that person. The rationales can be those that can be used for any client. The evaluation should determine whether the goals you listed have been realized. If all these guidelines are followed for one specific client, your care plan is individualized. (See two examples of individualized care plans in the appendix on Delmar's Web site and further discussion of component parts of the nursing process in Chapter 2.)

## KEY TERMS

**analyze**–To critically look at the component parts of the client data, determine their interrelatedness and their significance to the client's problems.

**assessment**–The beginning phase in the nursing process where patient data is collected. This forms the basis for the nursing diagnosis.

**caring**–An inner feeling of wanting to do, wanting to help. It is identifying with all the client's concerns.

**critical thinking**–Is an active thought process that analyzes all parts of a problem, arrives at specific goals to be realized, makes decisions about appropriate interventions, and examines outcomes.

**diagnosis**–The second phase of the nursing process in which the problems identified in the assessment are categorized from the NANDA approved list and named as present (actual) or likely to happen in a given situation (risk for).

**empathy**–In-depth understanding of a person's feelings and concerns and the ability to share warmth and understanding through verbal and nonverbal communication (giving of self).

**evaluation**–Examination that occurs throughout the nursing process to determine reliability of data, correctness of the nursing diagnosis, attainable goals, appropriate nursing interventions, and the realization of the expectations.

**goal**–A desired outcome.

**implementation**–The carrying out of the listed interventions (performing the required nursing care) in order to realize the identified client goals.

**interpersonal**–Relationship between people. Ways in which people interact with one another that may be positive or negative.

**interrelatedness**–The relationship between parts. Determining how each part affects the other.

**intervention**–Actions that are taken to treat or solve a problem.

**intrapersonal**–Looking into one's self to determine feelings and attitudes about others.

**intuition**–Quick and ready insight that, in some situations, might give one a feeling of impending danger.

**need**–A desire within an individual that, if left unfulfilled, can cause anxiety and stress.

**nursing process**–A systematic way of assessing, planning, diagnosing, and evaluating patient care situations.

**planning**–The phase of the nursing process where the assessment data and the nursing diagnosis are utilized in the formulation of client-centered goals and interventions in order to meet the client's needs. The health-care team and the client are actively involved in formulating the plan of care.

**prioritizing**–Sequencing according to importance. Arranging according to urgency.

## NURSING CHECKLIST

1. Prerequisites to developing a plan of care:
   - ☐ Review all the steps of the nursing process.
   - ☐ Ascertain what each step means.

- ☐ Understand that no step independent of the others can achieve client care goals/outcomes.
- ☐ Plan to follow the sequence as outlined:
  - assessment,
  - diagnosis
  - planning
  - implementation
  - evaluation

2. The nursing process is sequential.
   - ☐ Each steps builds on the preceding one.
   - ☐ If the first step is incorrect it is most likely the steps that follow will be incorrect.
   - ☐ To have a workable plan of care you must follow the following sequence:
     - assessment
     - diagnosis
     - planning
     - implementation
     - evaluation

3. Take action:
   - ☐ Assess the client—use assessment tools to collect all possible data.
   - ☐ Validate the data—reliable, relevant, past, present, subjective, objective.
   - ☐ Prioritize the data.

4. Evaluate the results: If your results are what you wanted to accomplish then your goals for the client are met. If they are not what you expected, rework the plan following all steps from the beginning and again work sequentially.
   - assessment
   - diagnosis
   - planning
   - intervention
   - evaluation

See completed care plan in the appendix on Delmar's Web site.

Formulate the Nursing Diagnosis:
- ☐ Check the NANDA list of nursing diagnoses.
- ☐ Look for the closest match to the prioritized piece of data (subjective, objective).
- ☐ Verify the nursing diagnosis with a list of defining characteristics for that specific nursing diagnosis (the one you selected).
- ☐ Write down the nursing diagnosis.

Plan
- ☐ Determine the outcome goals that you desire for your client.
- ☐ Plan how you will accomplish this by selecting nursing interventions from your nursing text.
- ☐ Implement the plan by performing the appropriate nursing skills.

Other points to remember
- The nursing process provides an organized format for planning client care.
- It is like a road map, which, if carefully followed, will bring you to your correct destination—that of helping the clients solve their problem.
- The process must begin with the assessment and follow in sequence: assessment, diagnosis, planning, intervention, and evaluation.
- You always evaluate your goals to determine whether they are met or not met.
- Never evaluate the interventions.
- If the goals are not met, it is likely they were unrealistic. Begin at the assessment phase again and rework the plan of care.
- Relook at the data. Ask if it is current, relevant, factual.
- Reexamine the nursing diagnosis (use the NANDA list).
- Reread the list of defining characteristics that pertain to your selected nursing diagnosis.
- Select at least three characteristics that correlate with the nursing diagnosis that you have chosen. This is to verify the correctness of your nursing diagnosis.
- Develop your critical thinking skills; that is, ponder what you are doing and ask questions of yourself: Is this right? Is this logical? Is this sequential? Is this relevant to this client at this time? Is this realistic? Is this individualized (how do I make this information usable to my client's situation)? Is this information generalized? Will the goals be realized (met)?

- Problem solve: Ask if this approach is followed, what will be the outcome?
- Make the decision to select the appropriate interventions that will enable you to realize a positive outcome (realize your goal).
- Use critical thinking to guide you into problem solving and decision making.
- Critical thinking must be used in all parts of the nursing care planning.
- Caring is intuitive, it is empathy that comes from within; it enables you to be patient, to use behaviors that help your client develop trust and confidence, and to reveal the inner feelings.

Always demonstrate a caring attitude.

- Communicate effectively; ask questions of your instructor and other nursing professionals; discuss your plans before implementing them. Develop good working relationships with others.
- Good client outcomes depend on good intrapersonal and good interpersonal relationships.

## CHAPTER SUMMARY

The nursing process is an organized plan of putting parts together in an organized whole. It helps you understand how to collect data and how to use the data to progress through the phases of nursing diagnosis, planning, intervention, and evaluation. The process also emphasizes the cyclical approach so you will know how to reassess and rework the plan when your goals are not met or new information must be incorporated. Critical thinking, problem solving, decision making, and caring are presented as invaluable components of the nursing process.

## REVIEW QUESTIONS

For each of the following, select the one best answer:

1. The nursing process is:
   a. A tool used to solve all clients' problems.
   b. A tool used to make inferences about clients' problems.
   c. An evaluation process used to determine student's performance.
   d. A way to teach test-taking skills.

2. Select the correct sequencing of the nursing process:

   a. Planning, evaluation, diagnosis, assessment.
   b. Assessment, planning, revision, evaluation.
   c. Reworking, assessment, diagnosis, planning, goal.
   d. Assessment, diagnosis, planning, implementation, evaluation.

3. How does each step relate to each other?

   a. Each step builds on the preceding one.
   b. The diagnosis relates to planning but not to assessment.
   c. The goal is the major part and leads to the evaluation.
   d. Relationship depends on whether the nursing diagnosis addresses an acute or chronic problem.

4. How does the nursing process facilitate nursing care planning?

   a. It helps to arrive at the nursing diagnosis with little or no effort.
   b. It provides a short pathway through the planning phase.
   c. It helps in data sharing among health-care personnel.
   d. It gives the social workers all the needed answers.

5. Which of the following is the best definition of critical thinking?

   a. It encourages analysis and differentiation of facts.
   b. It outlines only the nursing diagnosis trial and error.
   c. It is mainly trial and error.
   d. It is visible and interactive.

6. The purpose of decision making in the nursing process is to:

   a. Delineate actions that are needed, permissible, and correct.
   b. Convince the client to follow all orders as specified.
   c. Ascertain relief of pain.
   d. Prevent further hospitalization.

7. What is the purpose of problem solving in the nursing process?

   a. It provides tools for the nurse to use in solving the client's problems.
   b. It provides tools to assist the client in solving problems.
   c. It encourages each nurse to develop a new protocol for each client.
   d. It ascertains that all interventions are correct when first implemented.

8. Which statement best describes a caring attitude?

   a. A caring attitude is the determination to help the client recover.
   b. A caring attitude is the collecting of data from a wide variety of sources.

   c. A caring attitude is the nurse crying when the client cries and laughing when the client laughs.

   d. A caring attitude is the nurse allowing friends to visit as long as they wish.

9. Which of the following best describes ways of developing caring attitudes?

   a. Gaining insight into self and meeting clients' needs from a cultural perspective.

   b. Meeting client needs through group therapy.

   c. Convincing a client that an above knee amputation is the best therapy for a gangrenous foot.

   d. Not taking the client's vital signs because he does not desire to be awakened.

10. Which statement best describes good communication?

   a. Reading and rereading an order before implementation.

   b. Carrying out a verbal order (for pain medication) given by the RN team leader.

   c. Explaining in detail the client's problem to a family member.

   d. Directing all client's questions to the doctor.

11. One benefit of good communication is that it

   a. Assures rapid wound healing.

   b. Negates the need for spiritual support.

   c. Forms the basis for correct patient care decisions.

   d. Forms the basis for early discharge.

12. Which of the following is most likely to occur if the nurse fails to develop the plan of care sequentially and individualized?

   a. A positive outcome will result because trial and error most often works.

   b. Patient satisfaction will result because common sense is what most clients respect.

   c. A quick reunion with family will result because the real problem surfaced without going through the steps of the nursing process.

   d. Wrong nursing diagnosis, interventions, and outcome will result.

## ANSWERS TO CASE STUDIES

Critical Thinking (page 12)    1. F,  2. T,  3. T,  4. F,  5. F,
    6. F,  7. F,  8. F,  9. F,  10. F

Decision Making (page 14)    1. T,  2. T,  3. F,  4. N/A,  5. F,
    6. N/A,  7. F,  8. T,  9. F,  10. F

Problem Solving (page 15)    1. F,  2. F,  3. T,  4. T,  5. T,
    6. T,  7. T,  8. T,  9. T,  10. T

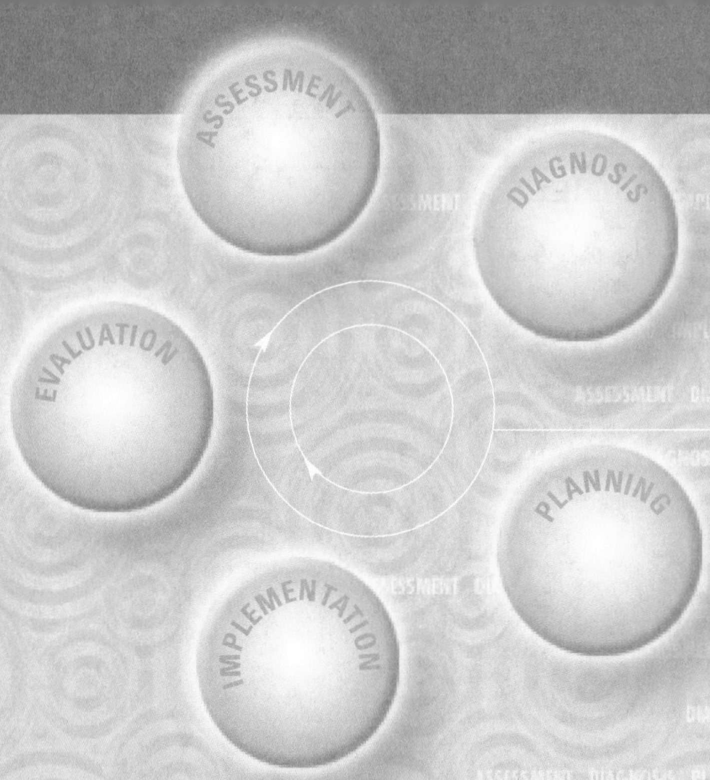
ASSESSMENT
DIAGNOSIS
PLANNING
IMPLEMENTATION
EVALUATION

## CHAPTER OUTLINE

# Assessment

## OBJECTIVES

Upon completion of this chapter, you should be able to:

- Define assessment.
- Discuss the importance of using critical thinking during assessment.
- Discuss the six major steps in data collection.
- Discuss how critical thinking relates to the pros and cons of data collection.
- Identify tools that contribute to comprehensive assessment.
- Differentiate between the interview and the physical assessment.
- Differentiate between objective and subjective data.
- Determine how information from the interview and the physical assessment are both crucial to validation of the data.
- Discuss an appropriate interview setting.
- Discuss the far-reaching effects of empathy and caring during the interview.
- Differentiate between closed and open-ended questions and their significance.
- State the rationale for the physical assessment.
- Discuss physical assessment from the Body Systems, Functional Health, Head-to-Toe, Human Response, and the Human Needs Patterns.

OBJECTIVES *continued*

- Discuss data analysis, data validation, and data clustering and their impact on the nursing diagnosis.
- Differentiate critical data that should be reported immediately from that which could be documented at a later date.

## KEY TERMS

| | | |
|---|---|---|
| assessment tools | focus | prioritizing |
| baseline data | interview | significant others |
| closed questions | open-ended questions | valid data |
| empathic listening | primary information | |

This chapter will provide answers to the reasons clients seek health care. It is designed to guide you through the various steps of data collection—revealing the sources from which to retrieve data, showing how to examine client data for relevance and reliability, and how to order data according to priority. The chapter also describes various assessment approaches that can be used to realize the goal of comprehensive individualized client care. The chapter emphasizes critical thinking, problem solving, and decision making. These active mental processes will guide you in selecting and organizing the data that are pertinent and significant. Detailed information on recording and reporting is also included.

## ASSESSMENT—WHAT IS IT?

Assessment is the initial step of the five phases of the nursing process. It is the collection of data that will enable you to think critically about the client's problems in order to make correct decisions about the plan of care. How do critical thinking and assessment interrelate? Assessment involves critical thinking.

You should think actively and intuitively as you question the client about incidents that caused the client to seek help from the health-care system. It is during the assessment that you take your first critical look at the client, intuitively searching for what is wrong and seeking out the problem. You think critically in order to determine whether there is one problem or many problems. The assessment must be detailed and comprehensive in order to facilitate identification of all problems. Through critical thinking you associate ideas and decide on the approach for collecting the data.

## Collecting the Data: A Critical Thinking Approach

You should begin by thinking about the various sources that you can use to collect information about your client. You should then organize these sources and follow them sequentially.

**Sources of Information**

Sources include the client, significant others, and medical records.

- The client—This includes what the client says about the existing situation.
- Significant others—From these individuals data is collected to confirm what the client says. The **significant others** may be family members and/or friends (see Figure 2–1).
- Medical records—The records (client's chart) generally contain many pages of information. You should read each page carefully. Think about what is significant and make notes. You are thinking critically about how each piece of information interrelates with all other information and how it impacts the treatment regimen. Examples are the physician's note on chief complaints, the medical diagnosis, orders that are written about the prescribed treatment, X rays and other diagnostic tests results, lab results, consultation advice, nursing documentation, and your literature review. Use the critical thinking process throughout your reading, determining factors that contributed to the medical problem and your goals for the plan of care.

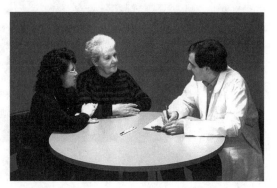

**FIGURE 2–1** Family members, such as adult children or spouses, can provide valuable assistance during the interview process.

### Steps in Collecting the Data

You will follow a sequence of steps when collecting data. The steps are:

1. Reviewing the client's chart
2. Interviewing the client
3. The physical assessment
4. Validating data
5. Clustering data
6. Focusing data

**Reviewing the Client's Chart.**   You may begin to collect your data by first reading the client's chart. This is advisable at the beginning of your clinical experience. This approach will provide a base from which to start the interview and the physical assessment. As you become more adept at data collecting, you may want to begin the process with the client and not the chart. This is likely to provide a greater challenge for you.

**Interviewing the Client.**   The **primary information** comes from what the patient says. You should listen attentively in order to gain the client's trust, which should facilitate disclosure. You will take notes during the interview to be sure you do not lose important information for the formal record to be completed following the interview (Figure 2–2).

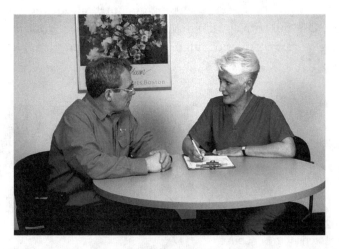

FIGURE 2–2   Write down important information during the interview, while maintaining your focus on the client.

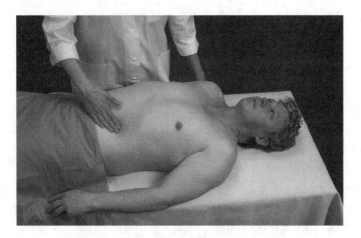

**FIGURE 2-3**  Technique of light palpation.

**The Physical Assessment.**    The physical assessment may begin before the interview is complete. This facilitates easy discourse during the examination and should help the client relax (Figure 2-3).

**Validating Data.**    You are to examine all the pieces of data that you have collected to make sure they correlate and they are accurate.

> EXAMPLE:   Validating the Data
>
> During the interview the client tells you that he has pain in his left side. On palpating the area he jumps and says, "Oh! That hurts." These findings would validate the data and would be accurate.

**Clustering Data.**    You now put together the pieces of the data that are similar. This will help you separate one problem from another.

> EXAMPLE:   Clustering
>
> Complaint of pain
> Demonstrated pain behavior

**Focusing Data.**    You should now look critically at each piece of data and draw initial conclusions and make tentative diagnoses.

EXAMPLE:    Tentative Diagnosis
Pain

## Collecting More Data

As you review your data, you may find that you are missing some basic information or that you need additional information to help you identify cause-and-effect relationships.

**Missing Information.**   If information seems to be missing in any pile of clustered data, you should attempt to fill in the gaps by asking further questions. This may be from the physician as he or she makes the rounds, from the physiotherapist during exercise, from the occupational therapist who provides assistive devices to aid in activities of daily living, or from family members.

**Cause-and-Effect Relationships.**   Now that you have acquired the data, you should begin to associate factors that might have created the client's problems and identify those things that might make it worse or better. You might have to ask further probing questions of the client and of family members. As you find these clues, you will work on a plan to decrease or prevent negative factors. You will sharpen your thinking as you study the pathophysiology of diseases. Questions you might ask are:

- Was there a relationship between his headache and his fall?
- Did his high blood sugar cause his headache?
- To what extent can he move his swollen knee?
- Should the knee be immobilized?
- Should the knee be cleaned and dressed before you perform your assessment?
- How severe is his pain and should he be given pain medication now?
- What about the high blood sugar? Should he be treated for this quickly?
- Why did his blood sugar get out of control and how do you help this?
- Can this client return to a high level of functioning?

## Prioritizing Data

Remember that some aspects of the data will reveal situations that must be dealt with immediately. You are to act on these promptly. If they are told to you during the interview or during the physical assessment, you would not complete your task before intervening. These may relate to reporting to someone with more expertise or may be as simple as adjusting the person's oxygen, repositioning a limb, giving the bedpan, or checking the IV site. Remember to pay attention to details. Data that is critical has first priority.

## Case Study

Mr. Simpson, 72 years old, was admitted with a fractured right femur. He has a Buck's traction with a weight of 10 pounds. He has slipped to the bottom of the bed. The weights are lying on the floor. He is screaming for the bedpan, the urinal, and also about his pain. You have come to do an interview and a physical assessment.

### TEST YOUR UNDERSTANDING

In what sequence would you perform your tasks in order to help this client? Mark one for first priority, two for second priority, and so on.

\_\_\_\_ Medicate for pain.

\_\_\_\_ Give the urinal.

\_\_\_\_ Perform the interview.

\_\_\_\_ Adjust the traction.

\_\_\_\_ Perform the physical assessment.

See answers at the end of chapter on page 79.

## Reporting Data

As you collect the data, some problems will require immediate reporting; for instance, a sharp sustained pain in the lower abdomen or a temperature of 102.8°Fahrenheit with a pulse rate of 110 and blood pressure of 170/110. These are emergency situations that require instant attention.

EXAMPLE:    Data Reporting

Mrs. Simpson, a 34-year-old client, was admitted with fever of unknown origin. The night nurse reported that at 0000 she had a temperature of 105°F. An hour after giving Tylenol her temperature was 98.8°F. At 0700 you find a temperature of 103°F. This finding should be reported immediately.

### Recording Data

Data are generally recorded at the end of the data collection period. There is often a data collection sheet where the protocol dictates what and how to record. You should follow these guidelines. Be sure to write legibly because team members often use this information for client status determination.

> **EXAMPLE:**    Data Recording
>
> Dr. XXX informed by RN. Tylenol 650 mg. Given PO as ordered. Stated he would see patient on his rounds.
> Signed: XXX Student Nurse

Validated, properly clustered, and accurately recorded data are likely to aid the finding of correct client-related problems. Inaccurate, invalid, and improperly recorded data are likely to result in wrong diagnoses and incorrect interventions.

## Tools for Comprehensive Assessment

**Assessment tools** are specially designed forms that provide a systematic and comprehensive way of collecting information about a patient in order to guide decisions about his or her care.

### Types of Assessment Tools

Some tools follow the medical model and resemble those used by physicians. They do not include specific information that relates to nursing. An example is the Body Systems Model. Other types of tools are developed to target nursing problems and medically oriented problems. They include nursing conceptual models such as Gordon's Functional Patterns Framework, Orem's Self Care Model, and Roy's Adaptation Model. Wellness models are also used (Kozier et al., 2000, pp. 99–101). You will most likely be exposed to one of these forms in your nursing program.

The form used in the clinical setting may be slightly different. Since most nursing care facilities use forms that relate to nursing, you should be able to make an easy transition from the form used in your class and clinicals (Figures 2–4, 2–5, and 2–6) to those used in other settings (Figure 2–7).

## Using the Nursing Assessment Tool

### Sequencing Data

You should carefully read each question on the assessment tool and follow the sequence from beginning to end.

**HEALTH HISTORY**

Name_____    Date_____    Time_____

**Demographic Data:**  Date of birth_____    Gender_____    Marital status_____

**Reason for Seeking Health Care:**_____
_____

**Perception of Health Status:**_____

**Previous Illness/Hospitalization/Surgeries:**_____
_____

**Client/Family Medical History:**

| | | |
|---|---|---|
| Addiction(drugs/alcohol)_____ | Diabetes_____ | Mental disorders_____ |
| Arthritis_____ | Heart disease_____ | Sickle cell anemia_____ |
| Cancer_____ | Hypertension_____ | Stroke_____ |
| Chronic lung disease_____ | Kidney disease_____ | Other_____ |

**Immunizations/Exposure to Communicable Disease:**_____
_____

**Allergies:**_____

**Home Medications:**_____
_____

**Developmental Level:**_____
_____

**Psychosocial History:**
Alcohol use:_____
Tobacco use:_____
Drug use:_____
Caffeine intake:_____

**Self-perception/Self-concept:**_____
_____

**Sociocultural History:**
Family structure_____
Role in family_____
Cultural/ethnic group_____
Occupation/work role_____
Relationships with others_____

**Activities of Daily Living:**
*Nutrition:*  Type of diet_____    Usual weight_____
Eating patterns_____
Types of snacks_____
Food likes/dislikes_____
Fluid intake:  Type_____    Amount_____
***Elimination (usual patterns):*** Urinary_____    Bowel_____
***Sleep/Rest:***
Usual sleep patterns_____
Relaxation techniques/patterns_____
***Activity/Exercise:***
Usual exercise patterns_____
Ability to perform self-care activities_____

**Review of Systems:**
**Respiratory**_____
**Circulatory**_____
**Integumentary**_____
**Musculoskeletal**_____
**Neurosensory**_____
**Reproductive/Sexuality**_____

**Health Maintenance Activities:**
Usual source of health care_____
Date of last exam(physical, dental, eye)_____
Other health maintenance activities_____

FIGURE 2–4    Sample assessment form: open ended.

# NORTH OAKS MEDICAL CENTER
## Initial Nursing Patient Assessment

| Admission Date | Room | Time |
|---|---|---|
| | | ___ AM ___ PM |

How admitted:    ☐ Ambulatory  ☐ Wheelchair  ☐ Stretcher  ☐ Ambulance  ☐ Other: _____

Accompanied by:    ☐ Family  ☐ Friend  ☐ Other: _____

| VITAL SIGNS | | | ORIENTATION | | | |
|---|---|---|---|---|---|---|
| Temperature | Height | | Call Light/Bed Control ☐ | Visitation Rules ☐ | Bed locked ☐ | |
| Pulse | Weight (Actual)) | lbs. | Television ☐ | Phone ☐ | | |
| Respiration | | | Educational Channels ☐ | Bathroom/Emergency Light ☐ | | |
| B/P | | | Lights ☐ | ID Band On ☐ | | |

### PERSONAL ESSENTIALS LIST / TRANSFER INFORMATION

| | | ☐ Sent Home | Date/Room | Date/Room | Date/Room | Date/Room |
|---|---|---|---|---|---|---|
| Valuables to Safe ☐ No  ☐ Yes (list on valuables envelope only) | | | | | | |
| Essentials at bedside: (check only those that apply) | | | | | | |
| Rings: ☐ Plain yellow metal  ☐ Yellow metal with stone  ☐ Plain white metal  ☐ White metal with stone | | | | | | |
| Watch – Describe | | | | | | |
| Hearing Aid  ☐ Left  ☐ Right | | | | | | |
| ☐ Eyeglasses  ☐ Contacts  ☐ Right  ☐ Left | | | | | | |
| Dentures  Full: ☐ Upper  ☐ Lower  Partial: ☐ Upper  ☐ Lower | | | | | | |
| Other (wheelchair, prosthesis, cane, etc.) | | | | | | |
| | | Admission | Sending RN | Sending RN | Sending RN | |
| | | | Receiving RN | Receiving RN | Receiving RN | |

### ALLERGIES

☐ No Known Allergies                    ☐ Yes

Allergy: _____    Type of Reaction: _____

| HEALTH PERCEPTION/HEALTH MANAGEMENT PATTERN | (May be completed by RN or LPN) | Nursing Diagnosis (Must be completed by RN) |
|---|---|---|
| 1. Informant:  ☐ Patient  ☐ Family Member  ☐ Friend  ☐ Unable to Obtain | | |
| 2. Present Illness/Current Complaint/Reason for Hospitalization: | | ☐ Health Maintenance. Altered  ☐ Noncompliance (Specify) |
| 3. Date last admitted to North Oaks Medical Center    ☐ Never admitted | | |
| 4. Previous Hospitalization/Surgical Procedures: | | ☐ Infection, Potential for  ☐ Injury, Potential for  ☐ Other (Specify) |

5. Medical History:
☐ Diabetes  ☐ Respiratory Disease  ☐ Cancer  ☐ Kidney Disease  ☐ Mental Illness
☐ Hypertension  ☐ Hepatitis  ☐ GI Disease  ☐ Thyroid Disease  ☐ Arthritis
☐ Heart Disease  ☐ Vision Disorder  ☐ Sickle Cell  ☐ Neuro-Muscular Disorders  ☐ Sexually Transmitted Disease
☐ Tuberculosis  ☐ Seizure Disorder  ☐ Blood Disorder  ☐ Problems with Anesthesia  ☐ Other:

6. Medications: Including OTC Drugs/Treatment Used at Home
☐ See Emergency Department Medication Review Sheet  ☐ List below if Patient not seen in Emergency Room

| Name | Dose/Frequency | Time Last Dose |
|---|---|---|
| | | |
| | | |
| | | |

Insulins: _____

Transdermals: _____

7. Do you take your medications as ordered?  ☐ Yes  ☐ No  Why? _____

8. Disposition of Medications:  ☐ Not Brought with Patient  ☐ Sent Home with Family  ☐ Sent to Pharmacy

9. Use of:  ☐ Alcohol  ☐ Tobacco  ☐ Recreational Drugs    ☐ Alcohol  ☐ Tobacco  ☐ Recreational Drugs
How Much _____  _____  _____  How Long _____  _____  _____

**FIGURE 2–5**    Sample assessment form: checklist. (Reprinted with permission from North Oaks Medical Center, Hammond, LA)

| SYSTEMS ASSESSMENT | (May be completed by RN or LPN) | Nursing Diagnosis (Must be completed by RN) |
|---|---|---|

**Cardio-vascular**
- ☐ Chest Pain  Rhythm: ☐ Regular  Radial ☐ Palpable  Dorsalis ☐ Palpable  Edema: ☐ Present
- ☐ Orthopnea  ☐ Irregular  Pulses: ☐ Non-palpable  Pedis: ☐ Non-palpable  ☐ Pitting
- ☐ Hypertension  Type: ☐ Pounding  ☐ Other  ☐ Other  ☐ Non-pitting
- ☐ Pacemaker  ☐ Thready  ☐ Absent
- ☐ Apical Pulse  ☐ Weak

**Respiratory**
- ☐ Cough  Chest ☐ Symmetrical  Breath ☐ Labored  Breath ☐ Clear all lobes
- ☐ Productive  Appearance: ☐ Asymmetrical  Pattern: ☐ Non-labored  Sounds: ☐ Equal & Bilateral
- ☐ Non-productive  ☐ Crackles
- ☐ Dyspnea  ☐ Rhonchi
- ☐ Orthopnea  ☐ Wheezes

**Cardiopulmonary**
** 1. Mobility Status: ☐ Ambulatory  ☐ Ambulatory with Assist  ☐ Bedrest  ☐ Transfer with Assist  ☐ Walker
2. Assistive Devices: ☐ None  ☐ Cane  ☐ Wheelchair  ☐ Crutches  ☐ Prosthesis  ☐ Pillows #_____
   ☐ Other _____
3. Limitations  ☐ None  ☐ Weakness  ☐ Fatigue  ☐ Other _____
_____
4. Do you have enough energy for desired activity?  ☐ Yes  ☐ No  Describe _____
5. Activities of Daily Living: I=Independent  A=Assist  D=Dependent
   ____ Feeding  ____ Bathing  ____ Grooming  Describe _____
   ____ Toileting  ____ Dressing  ____ Other

Nursing Diagnosis list:
- ☐ Activity Intolerance
- ☐ Airway Clearance. Ineffective
- ☐ Breathing Pattern. Ineffective
- ☐ Decreased Cardiac Output
- ☐ Activity Intolerance. Potential
- ☐ Gas Exchange Impaired
- ☐ Home Maintenance Management. Impaired
- ☐ Physical Mobility. Impaired
- ☐ Self Care Deficit (Specify)
- ☐ Other (Specify)

**Musculo-skeletal**
** ☐ Pain  ☐ Cramping  Muscle strength:  (S=Strong  W=Weak  N=None)
☐ Joint Stiffness  ☐ Spasms  Grips: ☐ Right ☐ Left
☐ Swelling  ☐ Tremors  Pushes: ☐ Right ☐ Left

**Neurological**
** ☐ Headache/Pain  Pupil Size: ☐ PERL  Level of ☐ Alert  Oriented to: ☐ Person
☐ Motor Disturbances  ☐ Other  Consciousness: ☐ Stuporous  ☐ Place
☐ Seizures  Right _____  ☐ Semicomatose  ☐ Time
☐ Numbness  Left _____  ☐ Comatose  ☐ Event
☐ Tingling  ☐ Combative
  ☐ Anxious
  ☐ Confused

** 1. Visual Impairment  ☐ None  ☐ Wears Glasses  4. Communication/Language Barrier: ☐ Yes  ☐ No
☐ Contacts  5. Level of Education:
☐ Blind ____Right ____Left  Grade _____
2. Hearing Impairment  ☐ None  ☐ Hard of Hearing  6. Pain/Discomfort:
☐ Deaf  ____Right ____Left  Describe: _____
☐ Uses Hearing Aid ____Right ____Left  A. Precipitating Factors:
3. Speech Impairment  Describe: _____
☐ None  ☐ Cannot Express
☐ Slurring  ☐ Cannot Understand  B. How is pain controlled?
☐ Mute  ☐ Tracheostomy  Describe: _____
☐ Stutters  ☐ Laryngectomy

Nursing Diagnosis list:
- ☐ Pain
- ☐ Pain Chronic
- ☐ Communication. Impaired Verbal
- ☐ Knowledge Deficit (Specify)
- ☐ Injury. Potential for
- ☐ Sensory/Perception. Altered (Specify)
- ☐ Thought Processes. Altered
- ☐ Unilateral Neglect
- ☐ Other (Specify) _____

**Integumentary**
☐ Normal  Temperature: ☐ Hot  Describe: ☐ Decubitus  ☐ Bruises
☐ Pale  ☐ Warm  ☐ Rashes  ☐ Scars
☐ Flushed  ☐ Cool  ☐ Wounds  ☐ None Visible
☐ Cyanotic  Turgor: ☐ Good  ☐ Lesions  ☐ Other
☐ Jaundiced  ☐ Fair
☐ Other  ☐ Poor
  ☐ Skin Intact

cm  1  2  3  4  5

**Nutritional / Metabolic**
1. Special Diet: ☐ Yes  ☐ No
   Describe: _____
2. Frequency of Meals:
   Describe: _____
3. Recent Changes in Appetite / Eating / Patterns?  ☐ Yes  ☐ No
   Describe: _____
_____
4. Have you experienced  ☐ Indigestion  ☐ Vomiting  ☐ Difficulty Chewing  ☐ Choking with Meals
   current/recent  ☐ Nausea  ☐ Sore Mouth  ☐ Difficulty Swallowing  ☐ Full Feeling in Throat
   Describe: _____
5. Recent Weight Loss/Gain?  ☐ Yes  ☐ No
   Describe: _____

Nursing Diagnosis list:
- ☐ Body Temperature. Potential Altered
- ☐ Fluid Volume Deficit
- ☐ Fluid Volume Excess
- ☐ Swallowing Impaired
- ☐ Infection. Potential for
- ☐ Nutrition. Less than Body Requirements. Altered
- ☐ Nutrition. More than Body Requirements. Altered
- ☐ Oral Mucous Membrane. Altered
- ☐ Skin Integrity. Impaired
- ☐ Skin Integrity. Potential Impaired
- ☐ Other (Specify)

| HEALTH PATTERNS ASSESSMENT | (May be completed by RN or LPN) | |
|---|---|---|

**Gastro-intestinal**
General  ☐ Well Nourished  Oral ☐ Dry  Bowel ☐ Present  ☐ Ostomies
Appearance: ☐ Malnourished  Mucosa: ☐ Moist  Sounds: ☐ Absent  ☐ Gastrostomy
☐ Obese  ☐ Nasogastric
  ☐ Jejunostomy

FIGURE 2–5  continued

**Patients At Risk to Develop Pressure Sores**  (May be completed by an LPN)

Identify any patient at risk to develop pressure sores by assessing the seven clinical condition parameters and assigning a score. Patients with intact skin, but scoring 8 or greater, should have the Nursing Diagnosis "Potential Impairment of Skin Integrity". Directions: Choose the number which best describes the patient's status. Total the seven numbers.

| Clinical Condition Parameters | Score | Clinical Condition Parameters | Score | Clinical Condition Parameters | Score |
|---|---|---|---|---|---|
| General physical condition (health problem)<br>Good (minor) — 0<br>Fair (major but stable) — 1<br>Poor (chronic/serious not stable) — 2 | | Mobility (extremities)<br>Full active range — 0<br>Limited movement with assistance — 2<br>Move only with assistance — 4<br>Immobile — 6 | | Skin/Tissue Status<br>Good (well nourished/skin intact) — 0<br>Fair (poorly nourished/skin intact) — 1<br>Poor (skin not intact) — 2 | |
| Level of Concsiousness (to commands)<br>Alert (responds readily) — 0<br>Lethargic (slow to respond) — 1<br>Semi-Comatose (responds only to verbal or painful stimuli) — 2<br>Comatose (no response to stimuli) — 3 | | Incontinence (bowel and/or bladder)<br>None — 0<br>Occasional (less than 2x in 24 hours) — 2<br>Usually (more than 2x in 24 hours) — 4<br>No Control — 6 | | Nutrition (for age and size)<br>Good (eats/drinks adequately - 3/4 of meal) — 0<br>Fair (eats/drinks inadequately – at least 1/2 meal) — 1<br>Poor (unable/refuses to eat/drink – less then 1/2 meal) — 2 | |
| Activity<br>Ambulant without assistance — 0<br>Ambulant with assistance — 2<br>Chairfast — 4<br>Bedfast — 6 | | | | Total | |

| HEALTH PATTERNS ASSESSMENT    (May be completed by RN or LPN) cont. | Nursing Diagnosis (Must be completed by RN) |
|---|---|
| **Genito-urinary**<br>Description per _____ Nurse _____ Patient<br><br>Urine Color: ☐Clear ☐Hematuria ☐Bladder Distention ☐Suprapubic Catheter<br>☐Dark ☐Cloudy ☐Foley Catheter ☐Urostomy<br>☐Other<br>☐Dialysis Access _____ | |
| **Elimination**<br>Description per _____ Nurse _____ Patient<br><br>1. Bowel: ☐No Problems ☐Diarrhea ☐Pain ☐Blood in stool<br>☐Constipation ☐Incontinence ☐Hemorrhoids ☐Other<br>Describe: _____<br>2. Bladder: ☐No Problems ☐Incontinence ☐Frequency ☐Burning ☐Nocturia<br>☐Retention ☐Dribbling ☐Dysuna ☐Urgency ☐Other<br>Describe: _____<br>3. Interventions: ☐None ☐Laxatives ☐Suppositories ☐Enemas ☐Other<br>Describe: _____ | ☐ Constipation<br>☐ Diarrhea<br>☐ Incontinence. Bowel<br>☐ Incontinence. Functional<br>☐ Incontinence. Total<br>☐ Urinary Elimination. Altered<br>☐ Urinary Retention<br>☐ Other (Specify) |
| **Reproductive**<br>Male ☐Penile Discharge ☐Pain ☐Inguinal Mass ☐Penile Implant ☐Other<br>☐Tenderness ☐Scrotal Mass ☐Breast Lumps ☐STD's (Sexual Transmitted Diseases)<br><br>Female LMP _____ Last Pap Smear _____ Pain with: Pregnant<br>Para _____ ☐Itching ☐Breast Lumps ☐Menstruation ☐Yes<br>Gravada _____ ☐Abnormal Bleeding ☐PMS ☐Intercourse ☐No<br>☐Contraceptive ☐Discharge ☐Other | ☐ Role Performance. Altered<br>☐ Sexual Dysfunction<br>☐ Sexuality Patterns. Altered<br>☐ Rape Trauma Syndrome<br>☐ Body Image Disturbance<br>☐ Other (Specify) |
| **Role Relationship**<br>1. Home Environment: ☐Lives with Spouse ☐Lives Alone ☐Lives with Family ☐Lives with Friend<br>2. Who do you rely on for emotional support? ☐Spouse ☐Family ☐Friend ☐Self ☐Other<br>Describe: _____<br>3. How does your illness/hospitalization affect your family/significant others?<br>Describe: _____ | ☐ Communication Impaired<br>☐ Verbal<br>☐ Family Processes. Altered<br>☐ Grieving, Anticipatory<br>☐ Parenting. Altered<br>☐ Social Interaction Impaired<br>☐ Social Isolation |
| **Coping/Stress**<br>1. Have you had any recent changes in your life (job, move, divorce, death, major surgeries, recent abuse)?<br>☐Yes ☐No Describe: _____<br>2. Do you feel you are dealing successfully with stresses associated with this change?<br>Describe: _____ | ☐ Violence. Potential for self-directed or directed toward others<br>☐ Role Performance. Altered<br>☐ Fear<br>☐ Other (Specify) |
| **Sleep/Rest**<br>1. Sleep: ☐No problem ☐Difficulty falling asleep ☐Difficulty staying asleep ☐Does not feel rested after sleep<br>Other _____<br>2. What helps you sleep? | ☐ Sleep Pattern Disturbance<br>☐ Other (Specify) |
| **Self Perception**<br>1. What concerns you most about your illness/hospitalization?<br>Describe: _____<br>2. Does your illness and/or hospitalization affect your sexuality/body image? ☐ Yes ☐ No | ☐ Anxiety<br>☐ Fear<br>☐ Powerlessness<br>☐ Self Esteem Disturbance<br>☐ Other (Specify) |
| **Values Beliefs**<br>1. Is religion important in your life? ☐ Yes ☐ No ☐ Religion/Faith _____<br>2. Do you have special religious request during this hospitalization? ☐ Yes ☐ No ☐ Notify Volunteer Services for Clergy<br>Describe: _____ | ☐ Spiritual Distress<br>☐ Other (Specify) |
| **Safety**<br>1. All areas with ** should be considered for FPP.<br>2. FPP should automatically be instituted for pts. who have/are: A) fallen previously<br>B) confused, disoriented or combative<br>C) chemical or physical restraints required | |

FIGURE 2–5   continued

**ADMISSION ASSESSMENT**

Date_____  Time_____

Admitted from:  Home____ER____Other____

Allergies_____

Baseline Data:  Ht____Wt____T____P____R____BP____

Mode of Transport:  Stretcher____W/C____Amb____

Home Meds:
_____    _____
_____    _____
_____    _____

| **Mental Status** | | | **Comment** |
|---|---|---|---|
| Alert/Oriented | Yes | No | _____ |
| Confused | Yes | No | _____ |
| Anxious | Yes | No | _____ |
| Comatose | Yes | No | _____ |
| Combative | Yes | No | _____ |

Other_____

| **Communication** | | | **Comment** |
|---|---|---|---|
| Speaks English | Yes | No | _____ |
| Aphasic | Yes | No | _____ |
| Speech Impediment | Yes | No | _____ |

| **Sensory** | | | **Comment** |
|---|---|---|---|
| Hearing Impaired | Yes | No | _____ |
| Visually Impaired | Yes | No | _____ |
| Amputation | Yes | No | _____ |
| Hemiplegia | Yes | No | _____ |
| Paraplegia | Yes | No | _____ |

**Diet/Nutrition**

Diet at Home_____

Likes/Dislikes_____

Appetite_____

| **Skin** | | | **Location** |
|---|---|---|---|
| Warm/Dry | Yes | No | _____ |
| Abrasions/Bruises | Yes | No | _____ |
| Laceration/Scar | Yes | No | _____ |
| Reddened Areas | Yes | No | _____ |
| Decubitus Ulcers | Yes | No | _____ |
| Burns | Yes | No | _____ |
| Rash/Scaling | Yes | No | _____ |
| Diaphoretic | Yes | No | _____ |

Other_____

| Color: | Pale | Normal | Cyanotic |
|---|---|---|---|

**Treatments in Progress**_____
_____
_____

| **Elimination** | | | **Comment** |
|---|---|---|---|
| GI:  Constipation | Yes | No | _____ |
| Frequency | Yes | No | _____ |
| Laxatives | Yes | No | _____ |

Other_____

| GU:  Frequency | Yes | No | _____ |
|---|---|---|---|
| Burning | Yes | No | _____ |
| Incontinent | Yes | No | _____ |

Other_____

| **Sleeping** | | | **Comment** |
|---|---|---|---|
| Unable to fall asleep | Yes | No | _____ |
| Awakens frequently | Yes | No | _____ |
| Sleep meds | Yes | No | _____ |
| Naps | Yes | No | _____ |

**ADL**                                   **Comment**

Assistance needed for:

| Ambulation | Yes | No | _____ |
|---|---|---|---|
| Eating | Yes | No | _____ |
| Bathing | Yes | No | _____ |
| Dressing | Yes | No | _____ |
| Eliminating | Yes | No | _____ |
| Turning | Yes | No | _____ |

Other_____

| **Denture** | Yes | No | _____ |
|---|---|---|---|
| **Glasses** | Yes | No | _____ |
| **Contact Lenses** | Yes | No | _____ |

**Personal Habits:**

| Tobacco use | Yes | No | _____ (quantity) |
|---|---|---|---|
| Alcohol use | Yes | No | _____ (quantity) |

**Chief Complaint:**_____
_____
_____

**Other Assessment Data:**_____
_____
_____

**FIGURE 2–6**  Sample assessment form: combination.

## Assessment in the Industrial Clinic

Following is an example of an occupational health history used in industrial settings.

I.  **Current Job:**

   A.  What is your current job title? _____

   B.  How long have you had this job?_____

   C.  What are specific tasks you perform on the job?_____
   _____
   _____

   D.  Are you exposed to any of the following on your present job?

   ___Chemicals          ___Infectious agents       ___Stress

   ___Dusts              ___Loud noise              ___Vapors, gases

   ___Extreme            ___Radiation               ___Vibrations
      temperature
      changes

   E.  Do you think you have any work-related health problems?

      If so, describe:_____

   F.  How would you describe your satisfaction with your job?

   ___Very satisfied  ___Satisfied   ___Somewhat satisfied   ___Dissatisfied   ___Very Dissatisfied

   G.  Have there been any recent changes in your job or work hours?

   H.  Do you use protective equipment/clothing on your job?

      If so, list items used:_____

II.  **Past Work Experience:**

   Please provide the following information, starting with your first job:

| Job Title | Dates Held | Brief description of job | Exposures | Injuries/Illnesses |
|-----------|-----------|--------------------------|-----------|--------------------|
|           |           |                          |           |                    |

**FIGURE 2–7**   Assessment in the industrial clinic.

## Baseline Data

**Baseline data** is a comprehensive assessment that deals with the client's problems from the head to the lower extremities at the time of first encounter. This should provide you with most of the relevant information that you need to arrive at the client's problem. You are also likely to find that the client's problem relates to one system more than the others. You should always follow this comprehensive format in data collection. You should now begin to focus.

## Focusing the Assessment

This deals with specific areas of the body. The problem may be localized and you should now **focus** on this area and collect in-depth information from interviewing and examination, including all related factors that pertain to the problem. This focused data prevents generalization. It narrows your focus for client care planning and zeros in on a particular problem. This enhances precision, efficiency, and client satisfaction, and is cost effective.

## Focused Assessment for Pain

As you assess for pain, you should ask a number of questions to gain a clear understanding of the client's pain—location, severity, and factors affecting the pain.

- Was there evidence that the client was having pain during the baseline data collection? Did the client admit to having pain? Was there a specific location for the pain? Was the pain described as sharp, dull, short-term, or persistent? How was the pain rated on a scale of one to ten, with one being least severe and ten being most severe?
- What factors relieve or aggravate the pain: rest, activity, positioning, eating, noise, quiet, medication, sleep, lack of sleep, daylight, night light?
- What measures need to be taken to relieve the client's pain?
- Is the client receptive to the treatment regime?

As you determine the answers, you will be able to choose specific relief measures.

## The Interview

The **interview** is the time you spend to hear the client's concept of the major concern and the reason help is being sought. This aspect of the interaction between you and the client is extremely important because you are seeking information that will substantiate the physical assessment. You will critically look at both pieces of information, the interview and the physical assessment, and draw conclusions about the care to be provided.

### Empathic Listening

**Empathic listening** is to listen with warmth and caring. It is the "giving of yourself." You must become intent on hearing what the client says. You need to avoid distractions and concentrate on the client. Allow freedom of expression; you should not change the subject while the client is speaking. You should demonstrate warmth and caring and actually assist the client in telling his or her story.

---

**Characteristics of Empathic Listening.**

- Sit at eye level.
- Maintain eye contact.
- Do not interrupt.
- Wait during a pause.
- Avoid long silences.
- Use repetition after a long pause if appropriate (observe nonverbal behavior).
- Use infrequent clarification to help the client listen to him- or herself and to affirm what you heard.
- Use mild confrontation to deal with incongruence in verbal and non-verbal communication.
- Show concern, warmth, and caring.
- Use touch when appropriate.

---

### Decision Making during the Interview

As you listen to the free flow of ideas you begin to put pieces of the information together. You start to draw conclusions and make decisions about problems that are of greatest concern to the client and the situations that need immediate attention. You also think of areas of concern that should be dealt with by other members of the team and make plans to communicate this at a later time.

### Carrying Out the Interview

You should select a place for the interview that is comfortable for both you and the client. This may be the client's room or some other place. A good temperature range is 65° to 78°F. You should help the client select clothing that will prevent chilling or overheating. Provide a comfortable chair or put the client in a comfortable position in bed. Remember to position both you and the client so that there can be good eye contact.

**Before Beginning.**

- Verify that you have the right client.
- Give your name and your credentials, and state your purpose.
- Set a time limit. Tell the client the interview should take about fifteen to thirty minutes.
- Observe privacy by closing the door and/or using a curtain.
- Do not rush and avoid interruptions. If you convey an attitude of haste, this may limit the information that is shared.
- Display confidence. Remember that you are likely to know more about this situation than the client and he or she will initially believe you know what you are doing. Demonstration of confidence will build trust.

**Asking the Questions.**   The questions you ask can be open ended or closed. **Open-ended questions** encourage the client to talk freely about problems. Because you give no strict guidelines or format, they are free to share and tell the whole story. Do not interrupt as long as the client is talking and remains on track. Remember to listen attentively so you can follow the trend of thoughts. If the client pauses, you are to wait and allow for the collection of thoughts. If the pause seems to be too long, repeat part of the client's sentence to help recall; for example, "You said you could not get off the floor." Be sure to observe the client's nonverbal communication. If grief is a factor, it may be so overwhelming that the client may need to wait before beginning again. Tactile communication (touch) may help at this time. If appropriate, you may place your hand on the client's body to convey caring and warmth. The following are examples of open-ended questions:

"Specifically what happened that made you come to the hospital?"
"If you had to explain this situation to a friend, what would you say?"
"Tell me what happens at night before and after you get into bed?"

**Closed questions** are also appropriate during the interview but are generally fewer than the open-ended questions. They are asked to get a pointed answer or a yes or no answer. A disadvantage of closed questions is that the interviewer may never get the total picture and many of the client's problems may never be identified. Examples of closed questions include:

> "Have you had breakfast?"
> "How many children do you have?"
> "Where is your pain?"
> "Did you fall at home?"

**Observing Nonverbal Behavior.**    You sit at eye level so you can note congruence or incongruence in the communication pattern. You may address these when appropriate. You may also save some of these for verification during the physical assessment. Here is an example of incongruence. You might ask the client, "How are you coping now that you have lost a leg?" The client answers, "I am coping very well. I am really not restricted in my activities." As you listen, you observe fear in the client's eyes and his face is flushed. An appropriate answer would be, "You seem to be suffering some hurt over this. There are tears in your eyes." Your statement would convey caring and should enhance the trusting relationship.

> **EXAMPLE:**    Congruence in Verbal and Nonverbal Communication
>
> "Nurse, I am so glad you came in. I feel exceptionally good today." The patient is smiling, demonstrates a "happy face." There is no evidence of tension and she communicates with the interviewer readily.

> **EXAMPLE:**    Incongruence in Verbal and Nonverbal Communication
>
> The nurse asks, "How are you today?" The patient answers, "Just fine, thank you."
>     The patient's face is flushed and tears are collecting in his eyes. His pulse rate is elevated.

**Recording the Interview.**    Your purpose is to listen attentively, not to write word for word what the client says. You should write down important points as the interview progresses. Do not ask the client to stop or to repeat a sentence so you can write it down. Remember to tell the client in advance that you will be taking a few notes to assist in the plan of care.

**Maintaining Confidentiality.**    Do not promise to keep a secret for the client. For example, during the interview the client may say, "I am going to tell you a secret. Promise me that you will not tell anyone." Your answer should be, "I will need to share all information that will be of benefit to the medical and nursing team in planning your care." Do not leave your written notes at the site of the interview. Remove the client's name from all your personal notes. Share information with other students only in conferences and with your instructor in private.

**Ending the Interview.**    Stay within the time limit (do not rush). Summarize the problems that you have identified. Ask the client to concur. Ask if there is anything else that should be added. You may ask for verbalization of the most urgent concern at this time. Determine if this is new information.

---

Sample Interview Session

Who: The student nurse and his or her client

Where: The client's room

Student: Good morning, Mr. Thomas. My name is Rebecca Marley and I am a nursing student from Ryan University. I am assigned to care for you today. I would like to take about half an hour to ask you some questions about your health. This will help us to give you the best possible care. This procedure is used with all patients when they are first admitted.

Client: That is fine with me. I will answer your questions to the best of my ability.

Student: What were the circumstances that made you decide to come to the hospital?

Client: I developed a severe pain in my belly this morning about an hour after breakfast. I started to vomit and it just didn't seem as if it wanted to stop, so I called a friend and he brought me to the emergency room, and here I am.

Student: Please tell me more about the vomiting.

Client: Well, I vomited about six times. Every time before the vomiting I felt like there were knots in my stomach and I would vomit a whole basin full. At first I thought it was blood but then I realized it was not that red.

Student: Can you think of anything the vomiting might be related to?

Client: I am really not sure, but I am wondering if it is food poisoning.

Student: Did you say food poisoning?

> Client: Yes, last night I had some leftover chicken and this morning I finished eating the chicken. It was about fifteen minutes after breakfast that I started feeling bad.
>
> Student: Tell me about the bad feeling.
>
> Client: I began to perspire, my head was spinning, and I got very weak, then the vomiting started.
>
> Student: How do you feel now?
>
> Client: I have never been this weak in my life. (Client's head falls back on the pillow involuntarily. His face is flushed and his pulse rate is 106 and respiration 30.) Right now I feel sick to my stomach but I do not have anything left in me to vomit.
>
> Student: Thank you for sharing this information with me. I will inform my instructor and the head nurse, and I will be right back to assist you.

The student nurse demonstrated the following appropriate behaviors during the client interview:

- Introduced herself.
- Stated her purpose for the interview.
- Set a time limit.
- Used open-ended questions.
- Allowed the client to speak freely without interruptions.
- Listened attentively, which is evident by her restatements.
- Looked for incongruencies.
- Ended the interview appropriately.
- Communicated her findings.
- Supported the client when needed.

## THE PHYSICAL ASSESSMENT

The physical assessment is a technique by which caregivers manipulate equipment in the examination of clients in order to find physical abnormalities in one or more systems of the body. It includes assessment of all body parts; for example, assessment of the pulse would be done at all pulse sites (Figure 2–8). It is done when the client is admitted to help identify existing conditions that will assist in diagnosis and the planning of care. It should also be ongoing in order to find new problems that might develop and that might result from the

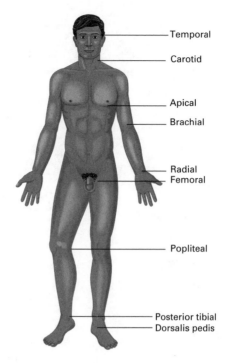

Temporal

Carotid

Apical

Brachial

Radial
Femoral

Popliteal

Posterior tibial
Dorsalis pedis

**FIGURE 2–8**  Peripheral pulse sites.

treatment regimen. The physical assessment also serves to substantiate findings from the interview. It may follow several approaches:

1. Body Systems approach
2. Functional Health Patterns approach
3. Head-to-Toe approach
4. Human Needs approach (Maslow's Hierarchy)
5. Human Response Patterns approach

## Assessment Using the Body Systems Model

The Body Systems Model is also known as the Medical Model and the Review of Systems Model, which focuses on anatomical structures of the body. When using this approach you should begin by assessing the patient's average state of health (general state of health). You then carefully assess the body systems sequentially: neurological, cardiovascular, respiratory, gastrointestinal, reproductive, endocrine, psychological and sociological, and family dynamics and relationships. (Medical Model has been modified by the author.)

Let us look at another example of the Body Systems Model.

## BODY SYSTEMS MODEL

| | |
|---|---|
| **Sensory Perceptual** | **Cardiovascular** |
| Mental status | Pulses |
| Hearing | Blood pressure |
| Vision | Capillary refill |
| Smell | **Neurological** |
| Taste | Orientation |
| Feeling | Pupillary response |
| **Skin** | Sensations |
| Color | **Gastrointestinal** |
| Lesions | Mouth and teeth |
| Edema | Bowel sounds |
| **Respiratory** | Distension |
| Breathing pattern | Swallowing |
| Breath sounds | **Genital** |
| Respiratory rate | Voiding pattern |
| | External genitalia |
| | Vaginal discharge |
| | **Musculoskeletal** |
| | Muscle tone mobility |
| | Range of motion |

*Source:*   Craven & Hirnle (2002). *Fundamentals of nursing: Human health and function.*
Philadelphia: Lippincott.

See the appendix on Delmar's Web site for an assessment and a fully developed care plan using the Body Systems approach.

## Assessment Using Functional Health Patterns

1. Health Perception/Health Management Pattern—The client's perception of his or her health status.
2. Nutritional/Metabolic Pattern—Relates to nutritional and fluid and electrolyte states, condition of skin and hair, height, and weight.
3. Elimination Pattern—The client's defecation and voiding pattern.
4. Activity and Exercise Pattern—relates to frequency of exercise and status of the circulatory and respiratory systems.
5. Sleep/Rest Pattern—Amount of sleep and rest and the effect on the client's body system.
6. Cognitive/Perceptual Pattern—Relates to the client's ability to hear, see, and taste; the perception of pain, smell, memory, speech, making decisions, and solving problems.

7. Self-Perception and Self-Concept Pattern—Relates to body image and self-confidence.

8. Role/Relationship Pattern—Relates to family dynamics and interactions.

9. Sexuality/Reproductive Pattern—Relates to satisfaction with sexuality and the sexual role and reproductive achievements.

10. Coping, Stress Tolerance Pattern—Stress management, self-management of stress, and the role of significant others in stress-related situations.

11. Value Belief Pattern—Relates to values the client cherishes and uses in decision-making and problem-solving situations.

12. Chief Complaint—The major symptom that caused the client to seek help.

13. Demographic Data—Age, sex, birthplace, religion, and place of residence.

14. General Appearance—Grooming and orientation, age, stature, motor activity, body and breath odors, dress, mood, speech, facial expression, and distress.

15. Past History—Previous health problems.

16. Family History—Illnesses in the family and causes of death of family members.

17. Vital Signs—Temperature, pulse, respiration, and blood pressure.

18. Measurements—Height, weight, temperature, pulse, respiration, and blood pressure.

19. Skin—Color, ecchymosis, lesions, temperature, texture, turgor, edema, and moisture.

20. Head and Face—Shape, distribution of hair, infestations, facial expression, symmetry. Eyes—vision; ears—hearing; nose and sinuses—potency, olfactory sense; mouth and throat—breath odor, buccal mucosa, teeth and tongue; taste—gag reflex.

21. Neck—Range of motion, trachea, carotid arteries, jugular vein, and lymph nodes.

22. Upper Extremities—Nail beds, capillary refill, muscle tone, range of motion, and pulse.

23. Back, Posterior and Lateral Thorax—Spine, lungs. Anterior Thorax—Symmetry, respiration, sputum, and lungs.

24. Heart—Cardiac landmarks and apical pulse.

25. Breasts—Inspection and palpation.

26. Abdomen—Inspection, palpation, and percussion.

27. Inguinal Area—Inspection and palpation.

28. Lower Extremities–Color, capillary refill, ulceration, hair distribution, varicose veins, temperature, edema, pulse, range of motion, and strength.
29. Neurological System–Mental status, orientation, and nerve responses.
30. Musculoskeletal–Mobility, range of motion, and scoliosis.
31. Female Genitalia, Anus, and Rectum–Pubic hair distribution, parasites, labia, urethral meatus, vagina, perineum, Skene's glands, and rectum.
32. Male Genitalia–Hair distribution, penis and scrotum, urethral meatus, and inguinal area.
33. Male Anus, Rectum, and Prostate–Perineum, sacrococcygeal area, and anal mucosa.
34. Psychological and Sociological
35. Health Maintenance Practices

Source: Estes (1998). *Health assessment and physical examination*. Albany: Delmar.

See the appendix on Delmar's Web site for an assessment and a fully developed Care Plan after the Functional Health pattern.

## Assessment Using the Head-to-Toe Model

When you are assessing using the Head-to-Toe format, you should first take the client's vital signs, and then assess the overall health. You should then assess all aspects of the patient's body beginning at the head and ending with the feet. Let us look at an example of the Head-to-Toe assessment.

### HEAD-TO-TOE MODEL

**Vital Signs**
General health
Temperature
Pulse, respiration
Height and weight

**General Appearance**
Color, orientation
Dress, grooming

**Mobility**
Posture
Ability to stand and walk—gait and balance
Ability to perform self-care—activities of daily living

**Skin, Hair, and Nails**
Hair quality and distribution
Skin turgor—wounds and abrasions
Nails

**Head, Face, and Neck**
Orientation
Memory
Speech
Hearing
Vision
Mouth and teeth
Cranial nerves

**Chest**
Inspection, auscultation
Palpation

continued

**Abdomen**
Inspect auscultation
Palpate quadrants
Liver, stomach, bladder
Elimination—bladder and bowel
**Genitalia**
Inspect male and female
**Extremities**
Inspect skin and nails
Assess pulse, reflexes, strength, joint
mobility, capillary refill, edema

*Source:*   Craven & Hirnle (2002). *Fundamentals of nursing: Human health and function.*
Philadelphia: Lippincott.

See the appendix on Delmar's Web site for an assessment and a fully developed Care Plan following the Head-to-Toe model.

## Assessment Using Human Needs Approach—Maslow's Hierarchy

When you collect data using these guidelines you will be looking at five areas as they relate to the client's needs. Let us look at these and their possible related problems.

| HUMAN NEEDS MODEL | |
|---|---|
| **Area of Need** | **Possible Related Problems** |
| Physiological | Comfort, warmth, food, fluids, elimination oxygen (adequacy of pain management, adequate diet) |
| Safety and security | Physical and psychological safety (unsafe environment, need for emotional support) |
| Love and belonging | Family and significant others (adequacy of support system) |
| Self-esteem | Pride and worthiness (need for building self-worth) |
| Self-actualization | Goal realization, self-fulfillment (identification of life accomplishments) |

See the appendix on Delmar's Web site for an assessment and a fully developed Care Plan using the Human Needs approach.

## Assessment Using Human Response Patterns

This assessment focuses on changes that are occurring in the client's nine response patterns and arriving at correct nursing diagnoses and nursing interventions to treat the problems. The response patterns are: exchanging, communicating, relating, valuing, choosing, moving, perceiving, knowing, and feeling. Let us look at each concept and a possible related problem and an example of nursing diagnosis.

### HUMAN RESPONSE PATTERN

| Concept | Relationship | Nursing Diagnosis |
| --- | --- | --- |
| Exchanging | Nutrition, elimination, circulation, oxygenation | Nutrition less than/more than body requirements |
| Communication | Sending messages | Impaired verbal communication |
| Relating | Family relationships | Altered sexuality |
| Valuing | Caring | Risk for spiritual distress |
| Choosing | Decision making | Ineffective coping |
| Moving | Activity, rest, activities of daily living | Self-care deficit |
| Perceiving | Self-concept | Hopelessness, powerlessness |
| Knowing | Information, cognizance | Knowledge deficit, impaired thought process |
| Feeling | Loss, sorrow, aggression, mental and physical distress | Pain, grieving, posttrauma response |

See the appendix on Delmar's Web site for an assessment and a fully developed Care Plan after the Human Response pattern.

## PERFORMING THE PHYSICAL ASSESSMENT

From the various models presented choose the model with which you are most comfortable or you may need to use the one selected by your instructor or the institution in which you are receiving your clinical experience. Regardless of the model, there are some basic things that you must do.

- Develop good communication between yourself and your client.
- Introduce yourself—"I am Pete Anderson, a student nurse from XYZ University."
- Give your reason for being in the room—"I am here to do a physical assessment in order to get information that will help us care for you."
- Secure privacy—Draw the curtains and close the door.
- Do appropriate portions of the interview while examining the client. This will help both you and the client decrease anxiety.

- Follow a systematic plan according to the model that you have chosen. By this you will display confidence and develop trust between you and the client.
- Jot information on your notepad. Remember to inform the client that you will be making notes.
- Answer questions truthfully.
- Avoid disruptions.
- Leave the client comfortable and safe at the end of the assessment.

## How to Develop Confidence in the Assessment Technique

Confidence comes with practice. Review the assessment tool and become familiar with the approach. Regardless of the approach, you will need to first determine the general condition of the patient and the reason for seeking care. That is the chief complaint. If an emergency situation exists, you will need to deal with this first. You will need to develop skill in these areas:

- Inspection—Looking at the client and describing what you see accurately.
- Auscultation—Listening for sounds through a stethoscope.
- Palpation—Feeling body parts to determine texture and consistency.
- Percussion—Tapping areas of the body and listening to resulting sounds.

The assessment tool you are using will guide you through the assessment. The Functional Health Pattern Tool, for example, will list questions about the eleven requirements, then deal with the chief complaint, the demographic data, the general appearance, the past history, the family history, vital signs, and on throughout all structures of the body ending with psychiatric problems of the client. The Head-to-Toe will begin with the vital signs, then assessment of the general appearance, mobility, and on throughout all the anatomical structures ending with the extremities. Remember to follow the sequence carefully to avoid frustration.

## Organizing Data

Now that you have collected the data, you will need to organize and validate the data. You should organize into groupings of subjective and objective information. Subjective information is what the patient tells you about the problem. Objective information relates to what you see in observation and what you find on physical assessment of the client in relationship to the client's verbalized statements. The subjective data helps you to critically look at the problem from the client's perspective. It also guides you to pinpoint what to look for and what to examine as you perform the physical assessment.

**Subjective Data**

The subjective data is beneficial to the caregiver in the following manner:

- Conveys the client's thoughts and feelings.
- Communicates the urgency of a situation in the client's own words.
- Statements accompanied by emotion give an idea of how severe the problem is from the client's perspective.
- Helps the examiner determine what to look for during the physical assessment. This is called making inference, what the patient says gives clues for observation during a physical assessment.
- Creates total acceptance of the client's statements or fosters further data collection for verification.

> **EXAMPLE:**    Subjective Statements
> "My arm is very painful at the IV site."
> "I am very sick to my stomach."
> "I feel very wet at my operation site."

**Objective Data**

Of what use is the objective data?

- It follows the ideas of the subjective data in physical assessment and observation to find the actual problem.
- It facilitates description and documentation of actual findings.
- It correlates with the subjective data to verify what the client states.
- Together with the subjective data it facilitates the formation of the nursing diagnosis and all subsequent parts of the care plan.

Let us look at the objective data that correlates with the previously written subjective data.

## ORGANIZING ASSESSMENT DATA

| Subjective Data | Objective Data |
| --- | --- |
| "My arm is very painful at the IV site." | Client demonstrates pain behavior. Brows are knitted. IV site shows redness with some bleeding. Intracath positioned at 35-degree angle. |
| "I am very sick to my stomach." | Client's face flushed and wet with perspiration. Suddenly vomits 200 cc of undigested food. |
| "I feel very wet at my operation site." | On examination, dressing is bloody and partially raised from incision site. |

Conflicting findings between the subjective data and the objective data prompts further data collection. Let us look at some examples:

| Subjective Data | Objective Data |
| --- | --- |
| "I have no appetite and cannot eat." | Client consistently gains weight every morning that he is weighed. (Doctor's order requires daily weight.) |
| "I cannot sleep at night. I need a sleeping pill." | Client falls asleep every night before the nurse passes night medications. |

The incongruence in both situations requires further data collection.

- **Situation One**—Assign one person to serve and pick up the client's tray and record the amount eaten. Determine whether the client leaves the unit to eat or eats food brought in by relatives. Findings will add to the database facilitating proper solution to the problem, or reassessment may uncover additional problems such as fluid retention.
- **Situation Two**—Confrontation may be necessary. Tell the client that he is asleep before the medications are administered. Collect data regarding the client's claim of insomnia. For instance, does he fall asleep easily but awaken frequently? Determine if the desire for a sedative is due to fear, habit, or other factors. Deal with the problem when the reason is found.

## Validating Data

**Valid data** is information that is correct and factual. Incorrect or invalid data will lead to the wrong nursing diagnosis, which in turn leads to wrong or inappropriate interventions. Hence, the purpose of validating is to confirm your information. You should always ask yourself if there is validity to what you have heard or what the patient tells you. Remember that you are making inferences, drawing conclusions that relate to the subjective data. For example, you enter the room and say, "Good morning, Mrs. Alport, and how are you today?" Mrs. Alport replies, "I am fine." You leave the room without observing the tears in the client's eyes. Later that morning you are told that the client was diagnosed with inoperable cancer of the ovary. If you had observed the cue of crying in spite of the verbal communication, "I am fine," you would have made an inference of "fear or grieving" and would have explored the situation further to determine the underlying cause. Why should you validate?

### Reasons for Validating

- Enables you to draw the right conclusions.
- Helps you focus on the specific area for physical examination.
- Helps to eliminate wrong impressions.
- Enhances further exploration and more data collection for verification.
- Can enhance a trusting relationship through empathic listening.
- Helps you identify the correct problems.

### How to Validate

The following points will help you develop good validation skills.

- Use only equipment that is in good working order while assessing the patient. (Thermometer, stethoscope, sphygmomanometers, scales, ophthalmoscopes, otoscopes.)
- Verify information told to you by others. Interview the client, read the chart, perform the physical assessment, correlate the information, compare and contrast and select the facts.
- Verify your own findings. For example, if the client appears older or younger than the age recorded on the chart ask the client to verify.
- Verify written information against your own findings. For example, if the client is scheduled for an amputation below the knee for gangrene of the right foot and you notice that the left foot is affected, report the matter immediately to your instructor and the charge nurse.
- Seek assistance when in doubt. For example, if a blood pressure seems too high or too low, ask your instructor to recheck after you have taken it a second time.
- Collect data from a variety of sources. When the subjective data do not provide adequate cues to enable you to make an inference or the information is insufficient, collect more data from the client's family and the laboratory and diagnostic findings.

- Determine congruence. Determine the match between what the client says and your objective data findings. For example, your client is a diabetic who receives insulin (70/30) every morning and every evening. He eats only 50 percent of his supper and states he is not hungry. Every morning his blood sugar is quite high. You should determine if there is food from another source.

## Clustering Data according to Relevance

When you interviewed your client you made notes (subjective data). When you performed the physical assessment you made notes (objective data). You also collected data from the client's chart and probably from the family. You are now to examine the pieces of data that correlate with one another; that is, match each subjective and objective piece of data with a corresponding portion. The reason you cluster the data is to arrive at the nursing diagnosis. All of the related portions should correspond to one diagnosis. It is like putting different colors of pencils together in a heap and then sorting them by colors and shades. You should also remember that you collected your data using an assessment tool and that much of this information was recorded on this tool.

We also discussed various models for assessment. The nursing models lend themselves well to formulating nursing diagnoses but the medical models also help us to identify problems of the various body systems. Now let us cluster selected assessment data according to several of these models.

---

**NURSING IN ACTION**

## Case Study—Assessment

**Client Data**

Mr. Harold Simpson was admitted on Sunday morning with a medical diagnosis of swollen right knee and diabetes.

**Subjective Data**

- Four children, ages 16, 14, 12, 10.
- Occupation—painter.
- Urinating about every two hours.
- Client states that he fell that morning from a ladder that slipped while he was painting the neighbor's house. He later developed a headache. He admits that he

*continues*

**Case Study—Assessment** *continued*

didn't sleep well the night before and he states that he is very upset because he was supposed to take his children to a basketball game that day. He says that he is agnostic but his wife and children are Protestants who go to church regularly and they are trying to convince him he should begin to attend church. He has had diabetes for 12 years, and sometimes forgets to take his insulin.

**Objective Data**

* Sex—male
* Height—5'10"
* Weight—160 lbs.
* T—98.6, P—100, R—30, BP—130/90
* Oriented × 3 (time, place, person)
* Skin warm and dry except in lower extremities
* Respiration increased
* Lungs clear bilaterally
* Abdomen nontender, soft
* Voided in urinal—300 cc and amber
* Blood sugar on admission—314
* Breath odorous (halitosis)
* Right knee swollen, bruised in several areas. Serosanguineous drainage—covered with white bath towel.
* Capillary refill more than 2 seconds
* Skin cool in both lower legs, pulse diminished in both legs
* Allergic to sulfa

**Assigning Portions of the Data Relating to Assessment Models: Functional Health Patterns**

* **Health perception–health management patterns:** diabetes for 12 years, sometimes forgets to take his insulin.
* **Nutritional–metabolic pattern:** Ht.—5'10", Wt.—160, T—98.6, P—100.
* **Elimination:** urinating every 2 hours. Voided 300 cc during the interview.
* **Activity–exercise pattern:** paints 5 days a week, no formal exercise pattern, extremities cool to touch, pulses diminished.
* **Cognitive–perceptual pattern:** oriented to time, place, and person.
* **Sleep–rest pattern:** didn't sleep well the night before. Severe headache just before the fall.
* **Self-perception, self-concept pattern:** sometimes forgets to take his insulin.

*continues*

**Case Study—Assessment** *continued*

- **Role-relationship pattern:** male, married, 4 children.
- **Sexuality–reproductive pattern:** married, 4 children.
- **Coping–stress tolerance pattern:** BP—130/90, P—100, R—30. Very upset because he had planned to take his children to the basketball game that day.
- **Value–belief pattern:** agnostic but was now planning to attend church with his wife. (See the appendix on Delmar's Web site for several Care Plans developed according to Functional Health Patterns.)

**Data according to Human Needs—Maslow's Hierarchy of Needs**
- **Physical:** male, age 40, Ht.—5'10", T—98.6, P—100, R—30, BP—130/90, lungs clear, severe headache, could not sleep night before, fell from ladder, bruised right knee, serosanguineous drainage, swollen, painful, voiding every 2 hours, voided 300 cc, eats 1200-calorie diabetic diet, capillary refill more than 2 seconds, pulse weak in lower extremities, allergic to sulfa.
- **Safety and security:** fall from ladder, severe headache, very upset because he had planned to take his children to the basketball game that day, was agnostic but had plans to start going to church with his wife.
- **Love and belonging:** married, has 4 children, very sad because he had planned to take his children to the basketball game that day, was planning to start going to church with his wife.
- **Self-esteem:** married, 4 children, occupation painter, had planned to start going to church with his wife.
- **Self-actualization:** occupation—painter. (See the appendix on Delmar's Web site for Care Plans developed according to Human Needs—Maslow's Hierarchy of Needs.)

**Data According to Body Systems**
- **Client profile:** 40 years old, male, Ht.—5'10", Wt.—160, T—98.6, P—100, R—30, BP—130/90, oriented to time, place, and person, diabetes for 12 years, allergic to sulfa.
- **Respiratory:** respiration—30, lungs clear on auscultation.
- **Cardiovascular system:** T—98.6, P—100, R—30, BP—130/90, lungs clear, capillary refill more than 2 seconds, pulse weak in lower extremities.
- **Nervous system:** oriented to time, place, and person, severe headache before the fall, pain in right knee.
- **Musculoskeletal:** right knee bruised and swollen, serosanguineous drainage from right knee.
- **Gastrointestinal:** always hungry; eats all the time.
- **Genitourinary:** voids about every 2 hours, voided 300 cc amber urine during the interview.
- **Integumentary:** bruises on right knee.

### Reporting the Data

Before you completed the assessment you might have found a problem that you reported to the charge nurse and that problem was addressed. For example, the client was short of breath. Oxygen was administered and he has $O_2$ by nasal cannula, is lying in a semi-Fowler's position, and is more comfortable. You have now completed the interview and the physical assessment. You probably have a sheet of paper with jotted notes. You should carefully read your notes and probably underline those situations that you realize are problems and should also be reported before recording. Other conditions of which you are unsure and in your mind are questionable should also be reported at this time. You might need to collect more data in order to give a thorough report.

### Reasons for Reporting

- Enables prompt treatment.
- Keeps all responsible individuals informed about existing problems.
- Facilitates further assessment by experts.
- Encourages collaboration among the health-care team members.
- Expedites the treatment and possibly the recovery period.
- Enhances your learning.

### How to Report Information

- Report only to members of the health-care team (keep all client information confidential).
- Report concerns promptly.
- Be explicit and complete. Describe the problem objectively; do not include what you think.
- Be sure to report on the correct client; identify the client by name.
- Include information that will help experts interpret the findings. For example, with a client who has vomited give the amount, color, time, frequency, and type of vomiting such as "projectile." Include the vital signs and occurrences that might have precipitated the vomiting and the client's condition afterwards.
- If the report is by telephone, state the place from which you are calling. Give a complete description of the client, including the diagnosis, and ask the receiver if they are aware of the person of whom you speak.

- It is a good idea to write down your information so you can follow a logical sequence when speaking face to face or over the telephone. Remember that beginning student nurses do not give or take orders over the telephone.

## Examples of Reporting

- **Good Report**—Mr. Simpson in room 420 vomited just after he ate his lunch. He had eaten 100% of the 1800-calorie low-fat diet. He vomited 300 cc of undigested food with streaks of blood. He was coughing and vomited during the cough. He is now diaphoretic. His vital signs are: T–97, P–110, R–32, BP–110/70.
- **Poor Report**—The gentleman in room 420 vomited what looks like blood. He is also wet from perspiration. It was during a cough that he vomited. He had just finished eating. His vital signs have changed. They are: T–97, P–110, R–32, BP–110/70.

## Recording the Data

It is very important that the baseline data be recorded. These are your findings of your first assessment of the client. They should be recorded as soon as possible after the assessment is complete. Points to remember when recording the data:

- Write legibly. Others need to be able to read what you have written. They may need this for information or to confirm further findings. You may also need to review them again when you are developing your plan of care. These notes may also be summoned in legal proceedings. Poorly written data may connote poor care.
- Always use ink. Most institutions use black ink. Remember to ask before beginning. The chart is a legal record that should be preserved for many years. Using a charting device that is easily erasable will affect the quality of the available information.
- If you mistakenly write information, do not erase. Draw one line through the information, write error, and initial. Then, write the correct information beside the error. Do not erase or obscure. This can be mistaken for disguise and substandard care.
- Chart objectively. Describe observations as they exist. Giving your own opinions is subjective and may be misleading.
- What you reported and to whom should also be charted and should state what was done to alleviate or improve the problem.

## KEY TERMS

**assessment tools**—Specific written guidelines (checklists) that guide the nurse in the comprehensive data collection from each client.

**baseline data**—Initial information gleaned from the client at the time of admission that facilitates the formulation of the medical diagnosis and the nursing diagnosis and confirms the need for further investigation such as laboratory and diagnostic tests and consultation from other experts.

**closed questions**—Questions posed by nurse to the client that generate yes and no answers. Should be used only for that intent.

**empathic listening**—Attentive listening. A posture maintained by the nurse throughout all client communication that makes the nurse cognizant of all that the client says. Empathic listening is verifiable by the nurse's restatement, confrontation, leading questions, and appropriate silence.

**focus**—The elimination of extraneous data and the pinpointing of the major factors that are causing the client's problem.

**interview**—A one-to-one relationship between the client and the nurse during which time information is collected and used to guide the physical assessment.

**open-ended questions**—Broad statements that encourage the client to explore and verbalize all feelings and concerns. These statements discourage yes and no answers.

**primary information**—Initial data collected from the client or significant others and verified by the physical assessment that leads to beginning nursing diagnosis or diagnoses and subsequently facilitates collaboration among the health care team.

**prioritizing**—Determining client's problems that require immediate action. Organizing problems and concerns on a continuum according to the immediacy of the need for intervention.

**significant others**—Individuals within the client's circle of family members, friends, or associates who have knowledge about past and/or current behaviors and are willing to share information or give other assistance during the client's illness.

**valid data**—Client information, which is substantiated by the client or significant other's verbal communication and the physical assessment.

## NURSING CHECKLIST

**Assessment**
- Client's Name–Medical Record Number
- Date
- Medical diagnosis
- Review of client's records
- Interview
- Identification of chief complaint
- Physical assessment
- Review of laboratory and diagnostic studies
- Validation of data
- Prioritizing of data
- Ordering of data
- Recording of data
- Reporting of significant findings
- Formulating of nursing diagnoses
- Planning of nursing care
  - Writing of goals
  - Listing of appropriate nursing interventions
  - Determination of scientific rationale

Other points to remember

- Quality nursing care depends on accurate assessment.
- Assessment tools provide guidelines for comprehensive assessment.
- Data should be collected from all available sources before developing the nursing care plan.
- Data should be validated before the nursing care plan is developed.
- Attentive listening during the interview will assist in development of a trusting relationship.
- Information from the interview serves to guide the physical assessment.
- Critical thinking and decision making serve to eliminate irrelevant data and aid in the formulation of correct diagnoses.
- Open-ended questions during the interview will encourage the client to share intimate feelings and concerns.

## CHAPTER SUMMARY

Assessment is the first step of the nursing process. It deals with data collection, data validation, data clustering, and data prioritizing. It focuses on two primary sections—the interview and the physical assessment—but depends on data from significant others and client's records for validation and reliability. The assessment data is the source for the nursing diagnosis. Data collection is an active intuitive process. It may utilize various health assessment profiles that have as a common goal holistic client-centered care.

## REVIEW QUESTIONS

Answer the following questions with **T** for true or **F** for false.

1. Assessment is the first phase of the nursing process.
2. Critical thinking is used in the assessment phase to make decisions about the best approach and to determine tools to be used to collect the data.
3. Focusing the data can only be done after all other steps of the data collection are complete.
4. The interview is of greater significance than the physical assessment.
5. For the collected data to be valid all the information from the various sources must correlate.
6. Critical thinking aids in sequencing of information in a proper time frame.
7. Data from significant others are used to confirm what the client says.
8. Diagnostic and laboratory tests are used to substantiate the medical diagnosis.
9. Assessment tools are designed to provide a convenient way to collect specific data on a comprehensive basis.
10. Information from the interview guides the focus for the physical assessment.
11. Client data are validated mainly from the physical assessment.
12. For a trusting relationship to develop between the nurse and the client significant others must be present during the interview.
13. When the nurse provides privacy and listens attentively, the client is more likely to share inner feelings.
14. Closed questions asked during an interview encourage examination and verbalization of the client's feelings.
15. The physical assessment provides objective information that validates or negates the client's complaints.
16. The major goal of the five different approaches that may be used for client assessment is to determine the client's problem/problems.
17. Any of the five approaches listed can be used by the nurse for client assessment unless otherwise specified by the caregiving institution.
18. Irrelevant data used to arrive at a nursing diagnosis always becomes relevant as client goal/goals are identified.

19. All data are of equal importance; hence, there is no client information that takes precedence when the nurse uses a caring approach.
20. Open-ended questions asked during an interview encourage examination and verbalization of feelings.

## ANSWERS TO CASE STUDY

Mr. Simpson (page 47) interventions according to priority

1. Give the urinal.
2. Medicate for pain.
3. Adjust the traction.
4. Perform the interview.
5. Perform the physical assessment.

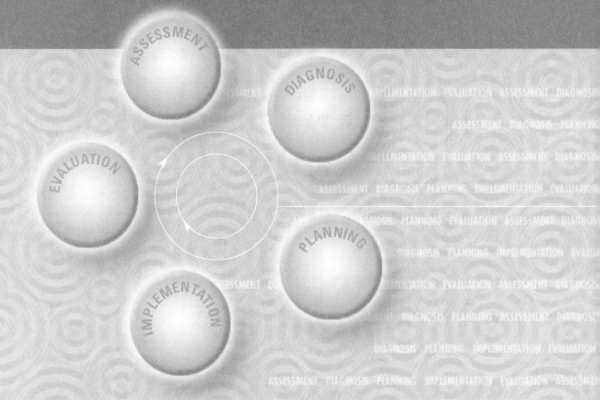

## CHAPTER OUTLINE

# Diagnosis

## OBJECTIVES

Upon completion of this chapter, you should be able to:

- Define nursing diagnosis.
- Discuss nursing diagnosis from a historical point of view.
- Relate nursing diagnosis to assessment and critical thinking.
- Identify the acceptable list of nursing diagnoses.
- Identify different types of nursing diagnoses.
- Differentiate nursing diagnoses from collaborative problems.
- Discuss the appropriate method for writing nursing diagnoses.
- Use critical thinking, problem solving, and decision making to select appropriate nursing diagnoses for client care situations.
- Use critical thinking, problem solving, and decision making to select data appropriate to each nursing diagnosis.

## KEY TERMS

actual nursing diagnosis
analyze
assessment
collaborative problem
defining characteristic
dependent nursing
function

diagnosis
etiology
independent nursing
function
ordering and selecting/
clustering

possible nursing
diagnosis
problem
risk nursing diagnosis
syndrome diagnosis
wellness diagnosis

In this chapter you will learn the meaning of nursing diagnosis and the historical contributions of nurses to this process. You will discover how to progress from the assessment to the next phase of the nursing process, the nursing diagnosis. You will find out how to select the correct nursing diagnoses and to differentiate between types of nursing diagnoses and collaborative problems. You will learn to appreciate how defining characteristics substantiate the nursing diagnoses. You will have the opportunity to use critical thinking, problem solving, and decision making in identifying relevant nursing diagnoses from client care situations.

## THE NURSING DIAGNOSIS: A CRITICAL ANALYSIS

What is nursing **diagnosis**? Identifying the nursing diagnosis is the second phase of the nursing process. The North American Nursing Diagnosis Association (NANDA) defines nursing diagnosis as:

A clinical judgment about individual, family or community responses to actual or potential health/life processes. Nursing diagnoses provide the basis for selection of nursing interventions to achieve outcomes for which the nurse is accountable.

If you examine the NANDA definition, you will find that in your previous **assessment** of clients' situations you discovered how they responded to changes in their health conditions. Now, if you apply a clinical judgment to these changes, you will actually be diagnosing. Remember that this list is already prepared for you. It is called the NANDA *Nursing Diagnoses: Definitions and Clarifications*. This leaves you to critically **analyze** the client responses in light of the various diagnoses in order to select the correct nursing diagnoses. The nursing diagnosis guides the planning of all nursing care and is the focus of all nursing interventions.

## HISTORICAL TIME LINE IN THE DEVELOPMENT OF NURSING DIAGNOSIS

Prior to 1950, nurses, for the most part, carried out physician's orders and were not autonomous. However, this began to change as highlighted below.

| | |
|---|---|
| **1950s** | Importance of nursing diagnosis discussed in nursing literature. |
| **1960s and 1970s** | Nursing theorists stressed the importance of problem identification by nurses with little success. |
| **1973** | Nurses initiated the development of nursing diagnoses in the First National Conference for the Classification of Nursing Diagnosis in St. Louis, Missouri.<br><br>The American Nurses Association endorsed NANDA in their publication *Standards for Nursing Practice* (ANA, 1973). |
| **1973–1991** | Nursing leaders continue to support nursing diagnosis in the nursing literature. ANA published *Nursing, a Social Policy Statement* (ANA, 1980) and *Standards of Clinical Practice* (ANA, 1991). The intent of these publications was to support nursing diagnosis as the second part of the nursing process. Figure 3–1 presents the ANA standard that relates to nursing diagnosis. |
| **1992** | Fifth Annual Conference of the organization renamed the North American Nursing Diagnosis Association (NANDA). |

<table>
<tr><td>

### ANA Standard II
### Diagnosis

The nurse analyzes the assessment in determining diagnoses. According to guidelines, the diagnosis must be:

* based on data collected during assessment of the client.

* validated with the client.

* documented so that it can be used in further development of the plan of care.

</td></tr>
</table>

**FIGURE 3–1**    Standard of clinical practice related to nursing diagnosis. [American Nurses Association. (1991). *Standards of clinical practice.* Washington, D.C.]

## TYPES OF NURSING DIAGNOSES

There are five types of nursing diagnoses: actual, risk, possible, syndrome, and wellness.

* **Actual nursing diagnosis** is a problem that is identified during the assessment. It is supported by obvious signs and symptoms. Examples are bathing/hygiene self-care deficit; dressing/grooming self-care deficit; feeding self-care deficit; and toileting self-care deficit.

* **Risk nursing diagnosis** is a problem that the nurse, through knowledge and experience, perceives will develop when risk factors exist. There are no signs and symptoms at this time, therefore, the words "evidenced by" would not be used. Instead, the words "related to" would be associated with the compromising situations in which the client finds him/herself. For example, all clients are likely to develop respiratory problems after a surgical intervention under general anesthesia. Nursing care will focus on preventing this problem. The nurse will write a diagnosis of "risk for altered breathing pattern" and "risk for altered respiratory function." Another example is "risk for constipation."

* **Possible nursing diagnosis** is a situation where data are insufficient to support or refute a nursing diagnosis until further evidence is gathered. The nurse may write a possible nursing diagnosis. One example is that of a person who lives alone and who provided his own home maintenance until this hospitalization. A medical diagnosis of "fractured right

hip" was made. The nurse may write a diagnosis of "possible impaired, home-maintenance management related to unknown etiology."

- **Syndrome diagnosis** is a diagnosis that is a part of a cluster of nursing diagnoses (Alfaro-LeFevre, 1998, p. 96). The two NANDA-accepted syndrome diagnoses are Risk for Disuse Syndrome and Rape Trauma Syndrome. Clients who suffer from long-term illness and are incapacitated are candidates for diagnoses associated with Risk for Disuse Syndrome. These diagnoses would be listed as "risk for powerlessness, risk for impaired body image, risk for social isolation, risk for impaired tissue integrity, risk for infection, risk for impaired mobility, risk for activity intolerance, risk for constipation, risk for injury, risk for altered respiratory status."
- **Wellness diagnosis** is a diagnosis that relates to a higher level of wellness for the client. There is no obvious problem. Nursing care would concentrate on helping the client maintain and achieve higher health status. Examples are "potential for enhanced parenting" and "potential for enhanced coping."

## ORDERING AND SELECTING THE DATA TO SUPPORT EACH NURSING DIAGNOSIS

Each nursing diagnosis will have supporting data. The process of **ordering and selecting/clustering** the data is critical to supporting the nursing diagnosis selected. Be sure to select the subjective and objective data that correlate and use these to select your nursing diagnosis.

## WRITING APPROPRIATE NURSING DIAGNOSES

When you write a nursing diagnosis you must include three components: the problem, the etiology, and the defining characteristics (Kozier et al., 2000, p. 292). The nursing diagnosis is also known as the **problem** or the diagnostic label. This is the specific client response to a health-related situation. You will find that one diagnosis may relate to several client responses in one given area. The word "specify" will be written against this diagnosis. Be sure to specify. For example, if the diagnosis is "self-care deficit (specify)," you will need to say if the deficit is feeding, bathing, grooming, and so on.

  **Etiology** gives the cause for the problem and is written as "related to" or "due to." More than one etiology may exist for one diagnosis. The etiology enables the plan of care to address the underlying cause of the problem. An example of a problem with its etiology is "altered skin integrity related to immobility."

**Defining characteristics** are specific signs and symptoms that must be present in order to confirm the specific nursing diagnosis as it is listed. More than one sign or symptom is required for confirmation. Defining characteristics are categorized as "major" and "minor." For confirmation of the nursing diagnosis the major characteristics must be present. The minor characteristics do not have to be present. The term "evidenced by" describes the sign and/or symptom that confirms the nursing diagnosis. An example is "Diarrhea related to gastrostomy feeding, evidenced by seven watery stools within 2 hours."

Risk diagnosis has no signs and symptoms; therefore, the words "evidenced by" would not be written. Instead, the words "related to" would be associated with the compromising situation in which the client finds him/herself. An example is "Risk for constipation related to restricted fluids."

## Case Study—Critical Thinking Relationship to Nursing Diagnosis

Always bear in mind that diagnosing involves critical thinking. Mr. Jones, a 75-year-old male, is admitted to the unit with a medical diagnosis of "lumbar pain." He states that "The pain started 2 days ago." He has been in a wheelchair for 1 year following a stroke. He has had a Foley catheter in place for 3 months because of incontinence. His urinary output is less than 30 cc per hour and is concentrated. He is being fed through a gastrostomy tube that has been in place for 6 months. He has one son who lives in Europe. He lost his wife a year ago. On admission his vital signs were: T—101, P—100, R—24. He wears a napkin, which shows no soiling on admission. He has lived in a nursing home for the past 6 months.

### TEST YOUR UNDERSTANDING

Test your critical thinking skills for the case study presented. Refer to the nursing diagnoses in Table 3–1. For items I–IX in the table, mark "True" for the nursing diagnosis and the related components if all parts are accurately stated. Answers to this exercise appear at the end of the chapter.

**TABLE 3-1**

Nursing Diagnosis Components

| | Nursing Diagnosis (Problem) | Evidence by (Defining Characteristics) | Related to (Etiology) |
|---|---|---|---|
| I | Acute Pain | Complains of pain | Aging—Change in bone structure |
| II | Impaired Mobility | Confinement to wheelchair | Stroke |
| III | Risk for Infection | | Invasive procedure—Foley catheter |
| IV | Altered Elimination | Urine less than 30 cc per hour—concentrated | Immobility |
| V | Possible Social Isolation | Needs more data | Altered family process Absent family member |
| VI | Possible Grief—Dysfunctional | Needs more data | Death of wife 1 year ago |
| VII | Hyperthermia | T = 101 | Unknown etiology |
| VIII | Risk for Constipation | | Immobility |
| IX | Risk for Disuse Syndrome | | Immobility |

Carpenito (2000). *Nursing diagnosis: Application to clinical practice*. Philadelphia: Lippincott, p. 387.

## WRITING COLLABORATIVE PROBLEMS

The **collaborative problem** is one that requires joint actions by the physician and the nurse. It is one where medical complications are likely to develop. The nurse performs **independent nursing functions**, interventions that are within the nursing scope of practice. **Dependent nursing functions** are those performed by the nurse in response to orders written by the physician when complications occur. Carpenito (1998) defines collaborative problems as "certain physiological complications that nurses monitor to detect onset or changes in status and should be labeled 'PC' (potential complications)." When you write a PC diagnosis, include the diagnostic statement and the likely complications. An example is "potential complications of pneumonia: hypertension, shock, respiratory failure, atelectasis, pleural effusion, delirium, and superinfection." (See Figure 3–2.)

| Disease/Situation | Complication (Related to) | Etiology |
|---|---|---|
| Potential complication of lung—pneumonia. | Hypertension, shock, respiratory failure, atelectasis, pleural effusion, delirium, and superinfection. | Inadequate drainage, insufficient blood supply to involved lung, and compromised immune system. |

**FIGURE 3–2**    Collaborative problem.

## WRITING NURSING DIAGNOSES THAT ADDRESS CULTURAL DIFFERENCES, ETHICAL ISSUES, AND SPIRITUAL CONCERNS

In the discussion about assessment, you were encouraged to deal with the client holistically. In other words, you must address all aspects of the client's needs and problems, including spiritual, ethical, and cultural considerations (Figure 3–3). Following the assessment, you must also address these three concepts in the writing of nursing diagnoses.

### Nursing Diagnoses for Cultural Needs

Nursing diagnoses that relate to culture include:

1. Noncompliance related to cultural beliefs
2. Knowledge deficit about the treatment regimen

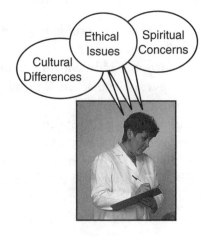

**FIGURE 3–3**    Always keep in mind that you must include an evaluation of spiritual, cultural, and ethical factors in the development of nursing diagnoses and the plan of care.

3. Risk for altered nutrition less than body requirements related to food idiosyncrasies

4. Risk for injury related to unfamiliar environment

5. Powerlessness related to perceived inability to change current situations

Examine the following client case study to identify the five potential problems (nursing diagnoses) in this portion of the assessment data.

## Case Study—Cultural, Ethical, and Spiritual Factors

Mrs. Martinez is a 70-year-old Hispanic client who has had diabetes for 5 years. For 4 years her blood sugar was controlled on oral hypoglycemics. Six months ago she sustained a bruise on her right great toe from wearing oversized shoes. This bruise became an open sore, which became infected "1 month ago." She used home remedies to treat the sore with no results. She visited an outpatient clinic where her blood sugar was 400. She was admitted to the general hospital where her blood sugar was regulated on Insulin Humalin Regular and on an 1800-calorie ADA diet. She was taught insulin administration of Lente 30 units (the dose on which she was discharged). She was readmitted with a blood sugar of 500 and a history of extreme drowsiness. The wound that had shown signs of healing now had a bloody discharge. During this interview she admitted not taking the insulin "because it is poisonous" and eating Mexican tortillas (her preference). She refused to eat the diet served in the hospital, stating "I would rather die than eat what you serve. Why can't my sister bring my food? I want to get out of here so I can cook tortillas." She was found wandering in her room late that night, and stated "I am looking for the bathroom. I am never left in a room by myself." She cried out "I have not seen my priest since you locked me in this place. I want him to be told everything about me."

### TEST YOUR UNDERSTANDING

From the information in the case study, cluster the data that relates to the following nursing diagnoses: Noncompliance, Knowledge Deficit, Risk for Altered Nutrition Less than Body Requirements, Risk for Injury, and Powerlessness. See answers to clustered data and corresponding nursing diagnoses at the end of the chapter.

## Nursing Diagnoses for Ethical Issues

Recall that in all aspects of the nursing process you are to apply your critical thinking, problem-solving, and decision-making skills. Therefore, during the assessment of the client you are to listen for statements indicative of ethical issues. You should make decisions on how to deal with these issues. Let us reexamine Mrs. Martinez's data for an ethical issue.

> **DATA:    CLIENT STATES:** "Tell my priest everything about me." If this request were granted, there would be a violation of the client's privacy since client data is confidential information. The nursing diagnosis for this problem could be written as Risk for Injury/Psychological.

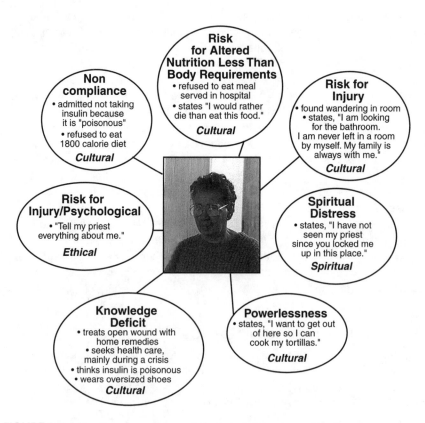

**FIGURE 3–4**    Nursing diagnoses and clustered data supporting the diagnoses.

## Nursing Diagnoses for Spiritual Concerns

Spiritual concerns should always be addressed during the assessment phase and related nursing diagnoses should be written according to findings in the data. Let us examine the spiritual concerns of Mrs. Martinez.

> **DATA:**  "I have not seen my priest since you locked me up in this place. I want him told everything about me."

Figure 3–4 depicts the cultural, ethical, and spiritual factors determined during the assessment of Mrs. Martinez.

## KEY TERMS

**actual nursing diagnosis**–A nursing diagnosis that displays specific signs and symptoms that relate to the client's problem.

**analyze**–Is to look critically at the selected data and the signs and symptoms it reveals and to determine the specific relationship to a particular NANDA diagnosis.

**assessment**–Relates to the data that you gather through the interview and the physical examination. It includes critical thinking, problem solving, and decision making in order to extrapolate that which is significant and reliable from that which is insignificant and unreliable.

**collaborative problem**–The nursing diagnosis that may develop and will require teamwork in order to arrive at client solutions. The treatment plan is not solely in the nurse's realm of practice, but the nurse carries out nursing interventions in collaboration with physicians and other health-care providers such as the dietician, social worker, occupational therapist, and physical therapist. Collaborative problems are written preceded with the letters "PC," for example, "PC pneumonia" meaning "potential for complication."

**defining characteristics**–These are actual signs and symptoms that are manifested when a client has a specific problem or disease. They are scientifically proven; hence, they are used to categorize specific problems and disease processes. Nurses use them to verify selected nursing diagnoses.

**dependent nursing functions**–Nursing interventions carried out in response to a physician's orders.

**diagnosis**–The nursing problem with which the client presents. It always relates to a specific portion of the client data and is chosen from the NANDA list of nursing diagnoses.

**etiology**–The factor that points out the cause for the problem/diagnosis.

**independent nursing functions**–The nursing interventions that are nurse specific. They do not necessarily need a physician's order. Most of them are scientifically proven to be effective when used to solve specific client care problems/diagnoses. They can be found in nursing textbooks.

**ordering and selecting/clustering**–Categorizing sections of client's data that correlate with one another. It includes what the client says during the interview (subjective data) and the signs that are found during the physical assessment (objective data). Both the subjective data and the objective data are ordered/clustered and used to determine the nursing diagnosis.

**possible nursing diagnosis**–Is written in a situation where the evidence for that problem did not exist prior to the client's accessing health care. However, because of the medical diagnosis, the possible problem/nursing diagnosis may develop.

**problem**–Another name for the nursing diagnosis. The terms may be used together; for example, nursing diagnosis (problem).

**risk nursing diagnosis**–Problems that a client might encounter because of diagnostic tests or other compromising situations of which the client may be subjected during the course of treatment, such as surgical interventions.

**syndrome diagnosis**–The term is used when the client has a chronic illness or suffers severe psychological trauma, either or both conditions may put the client at risk for many nursing diagnosis. These are written "at risk for."

**wellness diagnosis**–A diagnosis written when the client is not then complaining of symptoms of a disease and related signs are not evident. The objective is to assist the client to maintain or reach even a higher state of health or performance.

## NURSING CHECKLIST

**Diagnosis**

1. A prerequisite to writing the nursing diagnosis is to review all the data collected from the client.
2. Organize the data (subjective and objective components) that describe a problem.
3. Write all the possible problems–make a list. Include their corresponding data.
4. Look at the NANDA List of Nursing Diagnoses and select the one diagnosis that most closely matches the clustered data (think critically and analytically).

5. Examine a list of defining characteristics for that specific nursing diagnosis (the ones you have chosen).

6. Determine correlation between your ordered selected data and the signs and symptoms listed in the defining characteristics. See a list of some defining characteristics in the appendix on Delmar's Web site (signs and symptoms of some nursing diagnoses).

7. If you are able to, match at least three of these with your assessment data. You are seeing correlation between your assessment data and specific signs and symptoms (defining characteristics).

8. If the findings are the same in at least three instances, then it is most likely your selected nursing diagnosis is correct.

9. Include the three parts of a nursing diagnosis as appropriate—problem, etiology, and defining characteristics.

10. Differentiate between types of nursing diagnoses (write what you mean): actual, risk, possible, syndrome, and collaborative problem.

11. Critically look at the total list and put them in order of urgency (prioritize).

## CHAPTER SUMMARY

In this chapter, you studied the historical date line of the development of nursing diagnoses and were made to understand the commitment and importance that nursing leaders gave to this tool. They create a cluster of nursing problems/diagnoses to be used by nurses creating cohesiveness in the various parts of the nursing process. You were exposed to the various types of nursing diagnoses, and how they could be generated only as the assessment data is carefully analyzed, and ordered and selected (clustered). You were taught to write a specific nursing diagnosis only if it correlated with the specific defining characteristics (signs and symptoms) of that problem. The chapter emphasized that every formulation of a nursing diagnosis required critical thinking, problem solving, and decision making.

## REVIEW QUESTIONS

Select the one best answer:

1. The nursing diagnosis is supported by
   a. the defining characteristics.     c. planning.
   b. the goal.                          d. evaluation.

2. The nursing diagnosis relates

    a.  specifically to the medical diagnosis.
    b.  specifically to ordered selected data.
    c.  only to the interview.
    d.  only to the physical assessment.

3. How is an actual nursing diagnosis differentiated?

    a.  It is supported by signs and symptoms.
    b.  It has no etiology.
    c.  No signs or symptoms are evident.
    d.  It is always the first one recorded on the NANDA list.

4. What is the source of each nursing diagnosis?

    a.  *Index Medicus*        c.  NANDA list
    b.  *APA Manual*           d.  Medical dictionary

5. How does critical thinking relate to nursing diagnosis selection?

    a.  It focuses on relevant and significant data.
    b.  It focuses on irrelevant and insignificant data.
    c.  It avoids collaborative problems.
    d.  It avoids decision-making.

6. What is the best approach to selecting a nursing diagnosis?

    a.  Use critical thinking, problem solving, and decision making to select
        data appropriate to each nursing diagnosis.
    b.  Formulate the nursing diagnosis before beginning the assessment.
    c.  Always record what the client says as the priority diagnosis.
    d.  Remember that all risk diagnoses always become wellness diagnoses.

7. Syndrome diagnoses refers to

    a.  several diagnoses that relate to chronic illness or severe trauma.
    b.  medical diagnoses with unknown etiologies.
    c.  acute gastrointestinal disorder.
    d.  hyperpyrexia.

8. What is the classification for risk for diagnoses?

    a.  It already exists.
    b.  It is likely to develop.
    c.  It is always the priority problem.
    d.  It mostly relates to unknown etiology.

9. How is a possible nursing diagnosis classified?

   a. It already exists.
   b. It may develop because of a newly developed health problem.
   c. It was a diagnosis that was overlooked.
   d. It mostly relates to social isolation.

10. What is the best way to decide if a specific nursing diagnosis is right?

   a. Examine subjective and objective data and verify with defining characteristics.
   b. Select defining characteristics and match subjective and objective data with them.
   c. Show the client the list of NANDA nursing diagnoses and ask the client to select the one that relates to his or her problem.
   d. Ask family members to verify all relevant nursing diagnoses from a written list.

## ANSWERS TO NURSING IN ACTION: CASE STUDY— CRITICAL THINKING RELATIONSHIP TO NURSING DIAGNOSIS

I. T;  II. T;  III. T;  IV. T;  V. T;  VI. T;  VII. T;  VIII. T;  IX. T

## ANSWERS TO NURSING IN ACTION: CASE STUDY— CULTURAL, ETHICAL, AND SPIRITUAL FACTORS

| Clustered Data | Nursing Diagnosis |
| --- | --- |
| • Admitted not taking insulin, "poisonous" | Noncompliance |
| • Refused to eat 1800-calorie diet | |
| • Treats open wound with home remedies | Knowledge Deficit |
| • Seeks health care mainly during a crisis | |
| • Thinks insulin is "poisonous" | |
| • Wears oversized shoes | |
| • Refused to eat meals served in hospital | Risk for Altered Nutrition |
| • States "I would rather die than eat this food." | Less than Body Requirements |
| • Found wandering in room, stating "I am looking for the bathroom." | Risk for Injury |
| • States "I want to get out of here so I can cook my own food." | Powerlessness |

# CHAPTER OUTLINE

# Planning

## Objectives

Upon completion of this chapter, you should be able to:

* Define the term priority.
* Discuss the importance of priority setting.
* Discuss guidelines for priority setting.
* Define goals.
* Define outcome criteria.
* Explain the relationship between goals/outcome criteria and nursing diagnosis.
* Differentiate between short- and long-term goals.
* Discuss guidelines for writing goals/outcome criteria.
  1. Identify differences between teaching goals and discharge goals.
  2. Discuss the importance of writing cultural and spiritual goals.
  3. Relate standards of care to planning.
  4. Discuss legal and ethical considerations when writing goals/outcome criteria.
  5. Relate the various nursing standards to planning.
  6. Explain the sequencing of events when planning nursing care.

OBJECTIVES *continued*

7. Explain the rationale for recording the plan of care.

8. Analyze the component parts of a sample care plan.

9. Develop a plan of care.

## KEY TERMS

| | | |
|---|---|---|
| cultural/spiritual | long-term goals | short-term goals |
| discharge goals | outcome criteria | standards of care |
| goals | priority/prioritize | teaching goals |
| legal/ethical | recording | |
| considerations | sequencing | |

The planning phase of the nursing process follows the formation of the nursing diagnoses. The nursing diagnoses should be written in order of priority. This will lead to the goal determination and the selection of appropriate nursing interventions to meet these goals. In this phase, professional standards of care and the recording of the plan are addressed. **Cultural**, **spiritual**, and **ethical** issues as they relate to goals/outcome criteria are integral parts of planning and are addressed.

## PRIORITIZING

During the diagnosis phase you formulated many diagnoses. Some were: (1) actual (the signs and symptoms presented), (2) risk (where the application of the planned treatment could alter the client's state of health), and (3) collaborative problems (PC) (where the nurse cannot independently write prescriptions [nursing orders] and implement a plan of care). For collaborative problems, the nurse and the physician, and probably other members of the health-care team plan and implement the care. Look at your list of nursing diagnoses and **prioritize** them; that is, formulate each one in order of importance. Let us call this **sequencing** from most significant to least significant. Craven and Hirnle (2002) describe it as "something that takes precedence in position." This is done so that the problem that is causing the greatest danger, discomfort, or pain to the client can be addressed first.

It is good to number the problems (diagnoses) in numerical order, from one (highest priority), two, three, and so on to the least troublesome (lowest priority or problems that can be dealt with at a later time or referred). Remember that clients' priorities often change. Therefore, you must be aware of new developments and use your critical thinking, problem-solving, and decision-making skills to work with that problem that changed in **priority** from second to first place or from fourth to second.

## Case Study—Prioritizing

Mr. Bill Jones, 66 years old, had open reduction and internal fixation of his right hip on March 21. You are caring for him on his first postoperation day (postop). You read the nursing care for a client with this nursing diagnosis on the first postop day. You wrote and prioritized your diagnoses in the following order: (1) Risk for altered breathing pattern related to pooling of secretions related to general anesthesia, immobility, and reluctance to cough and use inspirometer. (2) Risk for pain related to surgical trauma. (3) Altered elimination related to relaxation of detrusor muscle due to immobility, decreased fluid intake, and general anesthesia. As you examine your client you realize his skin is warm and dry. On auscultation of his lungs you find no adventitious sounds. You are satisfied that the client's respiratory status is not compromised. You now decide to address your second priority, pain. The client admits to having pain. You are determining the location, the severity, and the nature of the pain when the client suddenly begins to vomit. You rapidly change your order of thinking. Your pain priority takes lower place on your list and you formulate the nursing diagnosis: Risk for aspiration of vomitus; client is lying with head of bed at 15-degrees elevation. You assist the client with an emesis basin, positioning, and other caring behaviors. You do further assessment to determine the cause of his vomiting. You report the incident, noting the contents of the vomitus, and then collaborate for further action. Always be aware of the need to change priorities.

### TEST YOUR UNDERSTANDING

Number the following nursing diagnoses from one through six according to priority (one is the most pressing and six is the least crucial).

* Ineffective breathing pattern related to hyperventilation evidenced by respirations of 50, and a radial pulse of 108.

* Ineffective airway clearance related to inability to cough effectively, evidenced by crackles and rales in base of lungs bilaterally.

* Pain related to trauma of surgery evidenced by guarding behavior and rating of pain as eight on a scale of one to ten, ten being greatest.

* Constipation related to habitual laxative consumption NPO day before surgery, day of surgery, and one day after surgery evidenced by no bowel movement for 5 days.

* Nutrition more than body requirements related to indiscriminate ingestion of food evidenced by 100 pounds above ideal body weight.

* Risk for altered skin integrity related to immobility evidenced by inability to turn self in bed.

**The answers can be found on page 126.**

# WRITING OUTCOME CRITERIA/GOALS

With the nursing process the terms outcome criteria and goals are often used interchangeably; however, there is a slight difference between the two terms. Let us define them. **Outcome criteria** is a specific expectation from the nursing intervention in the client care problem. The **goal** is a more general expectation that results from the intervention. The terms can be combined to show results from general to specific expectations; for example, the client will return to a normal bowel elimination pattern (general expectation) as evidenced by one soft bowel movement at least every other day (specific outcome). The terms will be used to show the general to specific in this book.

## Relationship between the Nursing Diagnosis and the Outcome Criteria/Goal

For every diagnosis that you identified, you should have an outcome criteria/goal. You should begin with the highest priority diagnoses and plan to treat them first. After you prioritize the problem you should ask "What do I want to happen for this client?" Your answer is your outcome criteria/goal. An outcome criteria/goal should have the specific components noted in the following list. An outcome criteria/goal is:

- Measurable
- Within time constraints
- Individualized to the client's needs
- Attainable/realistic

Goals should be written as short-term and long-term expectations.

### Short-Term Goals
**Short-term goals** can be realized within a short time. Sometimes the client situation requires a goal that should be realized within an hour or less. This will require quick thinking and decision making by the nurse. For example, a client experiencing tachypnea will need to control his or her breathing quickly. The goal, therefore, is very short term. Sometimes the outcome is controlled by the treatment protocol and the route of administration; for example, medications given by intravenous route should be effective almost immediately. The goal would identify relief within minutes. When medication is given intramuscularly, the goal would focus on relief within approximately 15 minutes. If medication is given orally, results could be as long as one-half to three-quarters of an hour.

## Long-Term Goals

**Long-term goals** are outcomes that will take a longer time to be realized. They may take weeks or months. They can also be written for shorter time periods. Because the nursing student is generally with the client for only two clinical days out of a week, it is good to write both short-term and long-term goals that can be realized during the period of interaction with the client. For example, if your clinical days are Mondays and Tuesdays, then aim at writing a goal that can be realized on Monday (short-term goal) and one that can be realized on Tuesday (long-term goal). There are many goals, however, that cannot be realized in two days. You should be careful to address these and collaborate with the nursing team to continue the regimen that you have begun. This will be to the benefit of the client even if you are no longer on the unit and therefore not able to evaluate the outcome.

## Measurable Goal

A measurable goal is one for which the outcome should be tangible, clearly visible, and of acceptable duration. A goal may be measurable both from an objective and a subjective standpoint. For an objective outcome, the results are observable and the client behavior or situation demonstrates change. Subjective outcomes are measured by the client's statements and confirmed by the corresponding nonverbal communication.

## Within Time Constraints

For each goal, a time limit is established within which the client can expect improvement. Each time constraint/limit supports the rationale for continuous assessment, thus facilitating documentation of outcome, further assessment, reporting, client and nurse satisfaction, and collaboration as needed for further interventions.

## Individualized to Client's Needs

All goals should be specific to the client—that is, to the overall client's needs—not merely to the medical diagnosis. You are to view the client holistically, realizing that the problems with which he or she presents are influenced or compounded by many factors, such as birth order; age; family relationship; economic status; work, living, and social environments; acute or chronic disease; the client's perception of the problem; and the coping ability. All of these factors will climax in forming the client's character, which influences the behavior that will be different from everyone else. Kozier et al. (2000) is in concert with this idea and writes that "dimensions of individuality include the person's total character, self identity and perception." When you formulate your goals, you are to use the general principles for writing goals, but you are to ask "Is this goal specific for this client and to what degree will it help the problem?" Ask what general principles need to be incorporated in order to realize the expected outcome. For example, the client's age is a factor in that you will likely formulate the goal for an adult differently from that for a child. Remember, a goal specific for one individual may not work for another. Let us examine a situation for specificity.

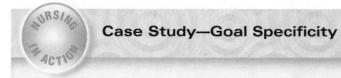

## Case Study—Goal Specificity

Mrs. Black is 60 years old. She suffered a stroke, which left her aphasic and with marked weakness of her left upper and lower extremities. This incident happened only the night before your encounter with the client. She lives alone in an apartment and is an only child. Both her parents died in an automobile accident three months ago. She worked in a women's clothing store. She made enough money to support herself but has no health insurance.

### Goals
After ascertaining that Mrs. Black is able to breathe adequately, it is reasonable that the next major goal would relate to communication. According to the general principles of goal writing, you should write: Client will communicate: (1) the circumstance surrounding the stroke, (2) the thing that gives her most concern at this point, and (3) things she would want the nurse to do for her, naming the sequence in which she would like these to be carried out. You would probably write that this would be accomplished between 0730 and 0800 (before breakfast). This goal would meet all the principles of goal writing: measurable, time specific, client centered, and realistic if Mrs. Black could talk. Since she cannot talk, the goal should be individualized to read:

### Individualized Goal
Client will communicate her immediate needs in writing (she is right handed and oriented to time, place, and person) between 0730 and 0800.

### Rationale
Client's health is probably too unstable for probing (may cause alteration in sleep and further damage to the central nervous system). It is important to gather all necessary information from the client but this should be done sequentially and determined by the client's state of health. Remember that individualizing takes critical thinking, problem-solving, and good decision-making skills.

## Case Study—Goal Specificity *continued*

**Attainable Realistic Goals**

Attainable and realistic means the goals should be set within parameters that can be reached by the client. The resources should be available to ascertain the expected outcome. Let's examine Mrs. Black's situation again. She is alert; oriented to time, place, and person; literate; and uses her right hand to write. She also suffered a stroke, which left her aphasic less than 24 hours ago. It is important that the client's most pressing needs (communication) be met; hence, the resources that are available to accomplish this are utilized—paper and pencil.

### TEST YOUR UNDERSTANDING

Write two short-term individualized goals using the following situation: Mr. Parks is 70 years old. He calls you to his room and states "I am bleeding." You find him standing in the bathroom with his clothes off, his incision from a laparotomy exposed (without dressing), and he is bleeding freely from the area. Suggested goals are listed below.

**Suggested Goals**

* Client will experience no further bleeding within 2–3 minutes (Monday, March 20).
* Client will maintain an infection-free state on Monday, March 20.
* Client will be injury free on Monday, March 20. The long-term goals could be the same for Tuesday, March 21. The client seems to be disoriented. Further assessment should be done.

## Examples of Short-Term Goals/Outcome Criteria

The following goals may be written for a client following surgery:

* The client will demonstrate effective breathing pattern between 0800 and 0830 on Monday, March 20, demonstrated by respirations between 18 and 20 per minute. Color will be pink and skin will be warm and dry (not diaphoretic).
* The client will verbalize comfort and rate pain as between one and two on a scale of one to 10 where 10 is greatest in no more than half an hour after pain assessment, evidenced by absence of nonverbal pain behavior (grimacing, guarding).
* The client's bladder will be nonpalpable within a maximum of 6 to 8 hours after surgery evidenced by denial of discomfort on palpation and denial of urge to void.
* The client will be free of physical injury between 0730 and 1500 on March 20, evidenced by absence of falls.

### Examples of Long-Term Goals/Outcome Criteria

- The client will demonstrate effective airway clearance by the second day after diagnosis of "airway clearance ineffective," evidenced by absence of adventitious sounds.
- By day three of surgery the client will require pain medication less frequently, evidenced by admission of comfort for prolonged periods of time and engagement in activities of daily living.
- The client will eliminate at least 30 cc of amber urine every hour by the second day after surgery having a total of not less than 240 ml in eight hours.
- The client will be injury free on March 20 and 21, evidenced by absence of falls.

### Teaching Goals

**Teaching goals** are similar to other client problem (nursing diagnosis) goals. That is, they should be time-sequenced, individualized, and measurable. They should most frequently relate to what the client needs to know about disease prevention, health promotion, health maintenance, and care. The goals should be written in the three teaching domains: psychomotor, cognitive, and affective. As you assess client data and formulate nursing diagnoses, you will realize that some problems relate to the clients' lack of knowledge about their disease conditions. This lack is called knowledge deficit and will relate to lack of knowledge in many areas. The goals should be written to correspond to the specific problem area. You should be careful to write them in all domains. Let us identify knowledge deficit problems in the following situation; then we will write teaching goals.

---

**TEST YOUR UNDERSTANDING**

Sarah Jane is 40 years old. She was admitted one day ago with a medical diagnosis of diabetes mellitus, type II. She weighs 210 pounds and is 5 feet 3 inches tall. She has an ulcer on her right big toe that is draining a small amount of serous-sanguineous fluid. Her blood sugar on admission was 490. She lives with her husband and four children, ages 9 through 15 years. She does not work outside of her home. She admits knowing about her diabetes 1 year ago when she visited the emergency room because of frequent voiding and headaches. She was given "pills for the sugar in her blood" and a diet plan at that time. "The pills lasted for 3 weeks but she was too busy with her husband and the children to return." She admits never having any diabetic teaching. The current doctor's orders read: warm compresses to affected toe twice a day, instructions on diabetic foot care, NPH insulin 30 units daily, regular insulin according to sliding scale, 1800-calorie diabetic diet (ADA). Client states she has always eaten what she wanted and did not discriminate between eating at night and eating during the day.

### Teaching Diagnosis
Knowledge deficit related to:

* dietary regimen
* medication and insulin regimen
* foot care
* exercise and rest
* home maintenance—delegation of duties

Think about the rationale (reason) for each of the following potential goals for this client.

### Teaching Goals
### Dietary Regimen
* Client will discuss the relationship of diet to diabetes (cognitive).
* Client will discuss the effects of ideal body weight on diabetes (cognitive).
* Client will write a list of foods that should be avoided on a diabetic diet (psychomotor).
* Client will write a list of foods she can use as substitutes in her diet (cognitive psychomotor).
* Client will state the benefits that she will realize from adhering to her diet (affective).

### Medication and Insulin Regimen
* Client will identify at least two types of insulin (cognitive).
* Client will discuss the difference in the actions of these two types of insulin (cognitive).
* Client will state the frequency with which her insulin should be administered (cognitive).
* Client will discuss the complications associated with excessive and too small amounts of insulin in the bloodstream (cognitive).
* Client will identify measures that she should take if she has a hypoglycemic or hyperglycemic attack (cognitive).
* Client will discuss the use of other medications to control diabetes (cognitive).
* Client will identify positive outcomes to self and family if the regimen is followed as prescribed (affective).
* Client will administer own insulin (psychomotor).

### Foot Care
* Client will discuss correct procedure for taking care of her feet (cognitive):
    Washing and drying
    Feet inspection

Reporting problems
Selecting shoes

* Client will demonstrate the proper dressing of the wound on her big toe (psychomotor).
* Client will state the benefits she will achieve from proper foot care (affective).

### Exercise and Rest

* Client will list at least three benefits of exercise and rest (psychomotor/cognitive).
* Client will discuss the relationship of exercise to excessive weight gain (cognitive).
* Client will develop and write a plan to exercise three times a week for at least 20 minutes each time (cognitive/psychomotor).
* Client will state the benefits of exercise to self and family (affective).

### Home Maintenance—Delegation of Duties

* Client will identify self as an important person (cognitive/affective).
* Client will discuss the benefits of delegation of duties (cognitive).
* Client will write out a plan for delegation of duties (psychomotor).

### Discharge Goals

**Discharge goals** relate to the expected achievements of the client during the regimen of care in the health-care setting and the level of expected performance in the client's new setting. Discharge goals should be contemplated from the time of admission. Like all other goals these must be individualized to the specific patient's needs.

Examples of discharge goals include the following:

* Client will state any feelings of inadequacy related to self-care in the home (cognitive).
* Client will state ways of getting help to solve problems that may occur after discharge (cognitive).
* Client will identify (list) physical hazards that will restrict activity in the home setting (cognitive/psychomotor).
* Client will discuss the treatment regimen to follow after discharge (cognitive).

## Planning the Nursing Interventions

After identifying the goals, you should now write the nursing interventions. Nursing interventions are actions that the nurse takes to help the client realize the specific goals/outcomes that are related to the various nursing diagnoses (the various identified problems). To arrive at the nursing diagnoses you asked "What is wrong with this client?" To arrive at the goals you asked "What do I want to happen in this person's behalf?" To arrive at the nursing interventions you should ask "What should I do to get the desired results for this client?" (achieve the goals). To get the answer to the interventions question you should use a reference that outlines specific actions for specific problems (diagnosis). You should remember to ask "Do these actions as written in this book apply to my client? Can I implement and use them as written or do I need to modify them for a closer fit to the existing problems?" You will need to have a good understanding of your client's limitations and the impact that the diagnosis or other problem is having on your client's health.

The nursing interventions should be approached in three different contexts: independent, dependent, and collaborative.

### Independent Nursing Interventions

Independent nursing interventions are actions that a nurse is permitted to perform independently. In other words, a physician's order or other professional's order is not required. You should become aware of actions that the nurse is allowed to do on an independent basis. These actions, however, should follow **standards of care** (see Standards of Professional Performance on page 114). It is best to write and implement independent actions before dependent and collaborative whenever possible. This will convey the autonomy and professionalism that nursing affords.

## GUIDELINES FOR WRITING INDEPENDENT NURSING INTERVENTIONS

- Use a good nursing reference.
- Be sure the action is permissible (does not require a physician's order).
- Ask if this action is applicable to this particular client.
- Will this intervention cause negative reaction of any kind? For example, types of soap for bathing or types of adhesive tape or areas of the body where vitals signs are prohibited, and feeding a client (withholding foods and fluids, making the client NPO).
- Ask if the intervention is still necessary since your previous assessment; determine the necessity of performing this intervention in sequence.

That is, if it is necessary to perform a first action and then a second, a third, and then the final and most significant action.
* Be sure the client clearly understands and agrees with the action.
* Determine the best time to carry out the action.

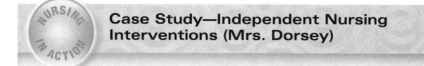

### Case Study—Independent Nursing Interventions (Mrs. Dorsey)

Mrs. Dorsey, age 36, is brought to the unit from the operating room after having an abdominal hysterectomy. The operation was performed under general anesthesia. She is awake but drowsy. You read in your nursing text that general anesthesia affects sensory, voluntary motor, reflex motor, and mental functions of the body (*Mosby's Medical Nursing and Allied Health Dictionary*, 2002). This means general anesthesia affects all organs and functions of the body. Mrs. Dorsey's drowsiness can be interpreted as a sign of anesthesia depression. The nurse is, therefore, required to monitor all systems until the patient is stabilized. As independent functions, the following should, therefore, be mentioned:

**Independently monitor:**
* Respiratory function—ability to breathe—and lung sounds
* Degree of oxygenation—color of skin
* Circulatory status—capillary refill and pulses
* Elimination—ability to void—bladder distension and urinary output if a Foley catheter is in place
* Neurological status—sensation to various extremities and degree of orientation and reaction of the 12 cranial nerves to stimulation
* Musculoskeletal—ability to move and reposition self, flexibility of extremities
* Pain—perception and severity of pain

### Dependent Nursing Interventions

Dependent nursing functions result from orders written by physicians for implementation by the nurse. As much as possible these should be done after the independent nursing interventions. Remember this is not always possible or advisable. The priority action may need to be dependent action. You should critically think this through and make the right decision. You should not blindly follow dependent nursing actions. Remember to ask if these are correctly written and feasible for your particular client. If your answer is no, then the written order should be discussed with the physician in light of your concerns.

## GUIDELINES FOR WRITING DEPENDENT NURSING INTERVENTIONS

- Be sure you have a written order for all actions that are not in the nurse's realm of independent practice.
- Read all orders at least three times and have a clear understanding of what the physician wants done.
- Check the rightness and feasibility of the orders for the client; for example, determine if the client is allergic to specific treatments.
- For medications, understand the dose, the route of administration, the duration, and the area to which the action should be applied.
- Determine the age-relatedness to the treatment.
- Know the frequency of application.
- Know potential side effects.

### Case Study—Dependent Nursing Interventions (Mrs. Dorsey)

The physician's orders read:

- Elevate head of bed only 45 degrees.
- Administer Demerol 75 mgm and Phenergan 25 mgm every 3 hours for pain.
- Ambulate after 6 hours.
- Remove Foley catheter in A.M.
- Keep NPO for 4 hours, then offer clear liquids and progress to soft.
- Change dressing after 24 hours.
- Give IV fluids of 5% Dextrose in 45 normal saline at 125 cc per hour.

After reading these orders you should implement them as ordered unless situations develop that prevent this action. These orders can be withheld if they are not feasible but there should be quick reporting to the physician about the action(s) taken by the nurse. That is, the nurse should report if there are reasons why the orders were not carried out as prescribed; for example, if the client had blood in the urine, you would refrain from removing the catheter until the physician had time to assess the new development.

**Collaborative Nursing Interventions**

Collaborative nursing interventions are nursing actions that require shared action by individuals from another discipline, such as the dietician, the respiratory therapist, the occupational therapist, the physical therapist, the speech therapist, the anesthetist, or the anesthesiologist. This commonly happens when information is to be given to a client and it is best given by an expert in that field. Although collaborative interventions can be an initial performance (a psychomotor skill), they are most often a teaching action in the cognitive and affective realm generally followed by a psychomotor action.

## GUIDELINES FOR WRITING COLLABORATIVE INTERVENTIONS

- Discuss client's needs with interdisciplinary team members when there are no specific doctor's orders and the needed interventions are not in the nurse's realm of independent practice.
- Determine the specific area of need and identify the person within the interdisciplinary team that can help to solve the client's problem.

### Case Study—Collaborative Nursing Interventions (Mrs. Dorsey)

Mrs. Dorsey has many dietary idiosyncrasies and she is also diabetic. Collaborate with the dietician regarding appropriate dietary changes for the client. Now that you have determined the various types of nursing interventions that are needed to solve the client's problems, you should record your plan.

## Recording the Plan

The plan serves several purposes:

- Provides in written format your goals for the client and the strategies (nursing interventions) that you plan to use to achieve these goals.
- Prevents duplication of work. It provides a base from which other nurses and other members of the interdisciplinary team can work.

- Identifies client care priorities. Problems are listed in descending order of importance, serving as a guide for nursing action.
- Prevents sensory overload—clients will not receive the same information on a repeated basis since resolution of specific problems will be listed in the documentation sequence and in a special column marked "resolved."
- Provides for more comprehensive care to the client. Documentation of resolved problems allows for the addition of more general problems such as health promotion and health maintenance.
- Enhances the client's rest and sleep patterns. There will be fewer interruptions with clear documentation of goal realization.
- Enhances trust relationship—all those who are involved in the client's care will be able to demonstrate adequate knowledge of the plan and the progression of care. This will build client–nurse confidence.
- Enhances significant other satisfaction. Adequate communication among team members establishes confidence.

**Recording** is often done on a care plan guide for the most part specific to the hospital in which you are receiving your experience. Sometimes your instructor will have a special chart form. This is generally adaptable to the one used in your clinical setting. Be sure to write clearly and legibly and sign your name after each category. See the example at the end of this chapter. The rationale for each written nursing intervention should be clearly stated and referenced. This is scientific data that you should select from a nursing reference text. The care plan documentation format should be sequential and logical and can proceed as follows: ordered and selected data, nursing diagnosis, goal (short- and long-term) interventions, rationale, and evaluation. The care plan will then be recorded in columns. Refer to the Nursing Care Plan at the end of this chapter. Recording should also identify the collaborative nursing diagnosis. Remember that you follow the same rule for collaborative nursing interventions when dealing with collaborative nursing diagnoses (independent, dependent, and collaborative) (Phipps et al., 1999). Refer to Table 4–1 for nursing interventions with rationales for a specific collaborative nursing diagnosis.

Other methods of recording the plan include SOAPI documentation and SOAPIER documentation.

## SOAPI Documentation
SOAPI is an acronym for subjective, objective, assessment, plan, and interventions. The planning of care may also be documented in this format. For example:
S—Client states "my feet hurt very badly."
O—Client is grimacing and face is flushed.

**TABLE 4–1**

Nursing Interventions for a Collaborative Nursing Diagnosis

| Collaborative Nursing Diagnosis | Independent Nursing Interventions | Rationale |
|---|---|---|
| PC: Pneumonia | Give oral fluids ad lib. | Helps to loosen secretions. |
| | **Dependent Nursing Interventions** | |
| | Administer O₂ as prescribed. Give medication as ordered. | Provides oxygen to tissues. Facilitates breathing. Serves as therapeutic regimen for specific conditions. |
| | **Collaborative Nursing Interventions** | |
| | Arrange with dietician to provide a diet that includes the four food groups and that is high in iron content. | Improves Hb and Hct blood levels and provides adequate nutrition. |

A–Right leg is swollen from toes to ankles (3+ edema). Visible necrotic area on right great toe–offensive; small amount serosanguineous drainage.

P–Short-term goal:

1. Client will verbalize comfort by rating pain at no more than two on a scale of one to ten within the next half an hour.
2. There will be absence of grimacing on the client's face (demonstrates comfort).

–Long-term goal:

1. Client will demonstrate comfort by requesting pain medication less frequently.
2. Edema will decrease to one to two plus by day two of treatment.

I–Interventions

–Independent:

1. Place leg in position of comfort.
2. Assess pain on a scale of one to ten, with ten being greatest.
3. Have client identify measures previously used successfully for pain relief.
4. Discuss pain measures prescribed by physician.

–Dependent: Administer treatment as ordered by physician

–Collaborative: If ordered treatment is ineffective, collaborate with physician for an alternative.

## SOAPIER Documentation

SOAPIER is the acronym for subjective, objective, assessment, intervention, evaluation, and reassessment. For example:

S–Client states "I am very nauseated and just vomited my lunch."

O–1. Client's face is flushed.

2. Emesis basin on bed with 150 cc of undigested food.

A–Abdomen is soft; bowel sounds are absent in all four quadrants.

P– 1. Short-term goal: Client will deny nausea within half an hour of assessment.

2. Client will state reason for remaining NPO for next 1 to 2 hours.

3. Long-term goal: Client will continue to deny nausea. There will be no further vomiting within the next 4 hours from assessment.

I–Independent:

1. Explain the relationship between active bowel sounds (peristalsis) and digestion.

2. Explain the possible reason for vomiting.

3. Discuss the benefit of the NPO state.

4. Encourage client to take deep breaths through the mouth when nauseated.

–Dependent: Administer antiemetic medication as ordered.

–Collaborative:

1. Ask dietary department to hold client's tray until further orders.

2. Collaborate with physician for another antiemetic if first order is ineffective.

E–Client states she felt she might have eaten too soon and too much. Agreed to wait until she was given the "all clear." Admitted feeling less nauseated after Phenergan 25 mg was administered. Denied nausea at supper time. Had clear liquid supper. Goal met.

R–If the goals were not met, you should reassess to determine the true nature of the problem.

## APPLYING STANDARDS OF CARE TO NURSING PROCESS

The component parts of the nursing process that we have discussed were identified and regulated by the American Nurses Association, which is the national professional organization for nursing in the United States. Before working with either component of the nursing process, you need to become familiar with the guidelines set by this organization in order to maintain the high standards of nursing practice that they require and to become aware that all nurses are required to follow these standards.

## Standards of Care

**I. Assessment**
The nurse collects patient health data.

**II. Diagnosis**
The nurse analyzes the assessment data in determining diagnosis.

---

### ANA Standards of Professional Performance

I. Quality of Care
The nurse systematically evaluates the quality and effectiveness of nursing practice.

II. Performance Appraisal
The nurse evaluates his or her own nursing practice in relation to professional practice standards and relevant statutes and regulations.

III. Education
The nurse acquires and maintains correct knowledge in nursing practice.

IV. Collegiality
The nurse interacts with and contributes to the professional development of peers and other health-care providers as colleagues.

V. Ethics
The nurse's decisions and actions on behalf of patient are determined in an ethical manner.

VI. Collaboration
The nurse collaborates with the patient, family and other health-care providers in providing patient care.

VII. Research
The nurse uses research findings in practice.

VIII. Resource Utilization
The nurse considers factors related to safety effectiveness and cost in planning and delivering patient care.

---

**FIGURE 4–1** ANA Standards of Professional Performance. (Reprinted with permission from American Nurses Foundation/American Nurses Association, 600 Maryland Avenue SW, Suite 100W, Washington, D.C. 20024-25710)

III. **Outcome Identification**

The nurse identifies expected outcomes and individualizes these to the patient.

IV. **Planning**

The nurse develops a plan of care that prescribes interventions to attain expected outcomes.

V. **Implementation**

The nurse implements the interventions identified in the plan of care.

VI. **Evaluation**

The nurse evaluates the patient's progress toward the attainment of outcomes.

**Utilizing Nursing Standards in the Delivery of Client Care**

Although nurses practice autonomously (as in the case of independent functions during nursing interventions), all nursing practice is regulated by nurse practice acts of the various states in the United States. These must be clearly adhered to as you provide independent, dependent, and collaborative care to clients. Let us examine the ANA Standards of Professional Performance (Figure 4–1).

## ETHICAL, LEGAL, CULTURAL, AND SPIRITUAL CONSIDERATIONS WHEN WRITING OUTCOME CRITERIA/GOALS

In writing outcome criteria the nurse needs to be attentive to ethical and **legal** responsibilities, as well as cultural and spiritual factors.

### Ethical Considerations

The nurse needs to be aware that ethics relate to morality and that clients' moral behavior is acquired over time and influenced by societal norms, family interactions, and group practice. The intent of nursing is not to change the client's moral thinking but rather to provide care in a nonjudgmental manner. This can be done according to ANA Standard V of Professional Performance. The nurse's decisions and actions on behalf of clients are determined in an ethical manner. This is measured by specific criteria (see Figure 4–2).

Let us now write corresponding goals/outcomes for the ethical issues diagnoses that were written in Chapter 3. See Table 4–2.

---

### Measurement Criteria

1. The nurse's practice is guided by the Code for Nurses.

2. The nurse maintains patient's confidentiality within legal and regulatory parameters.

3. The nurse acts as a patient advocate and assists patients in developing skills so they can advocate for themselves.

4. The nurse delivers care in a manner that preserves patient autonomy, dignity, and rights.

5. The nurse delivers care in a nonjudgmental and nondiscriminatory manner that is sensitive to patient diversity.

6. The nurse seeks available resources in formulating ethical decisions.

---

**FIGURE 4–2**   Measurement criteria for ethical decision making. (Reprinted with permission from American Nurses Association, *Standards of clinical practice* (2nd ed.). Washington, D.C.: Author, 1998, pp. 13–14)

## Legal Considerations

The planning and writing of goals should be a cooperative effort between the client and the nurse. This refers to the professional nurse as well as the student. This approach aims at preventing legal problems in all aspects of the care you provide. Remember that you can be held liable for all your actions, independent, dependent, and collaborative. Look at these examples: (1) The nurse gives an antihypertensive medication without checking the client's blood pressure (independent function) after the client complained of dizziness. Subsequently the client falls on ambulation and sustains a hip fracture. (2) The nurse administers penicillin as ordered by the physician without assessing the client for allergies. As a result, the client develops anaphylactic shock. (3) The nurse arranges alternate food choices with the dietician without identifying food idiosyncrasies with the client. As a result, there is anger and frustration and

| TABLE 4–2 | | |
|---|---|---|
| **Nursing Diagnosis and Corresponding Goals for Meeting Ethical Issues** | | |
| **Nursing Diagnosis** | **Short-Term Goals** | **Long-Term Goals** |
| **Risk for Injury Psychosocial** | • Client will verbalize understanding of confidentiality of client information. | • Client will be free of psychological trauma related to slander (exposure of confidential information). |

the client leaves the care setting prematurely against medical advice and falls while walking down the stairs. All three incidents can be labeled negligence and/or malpractice.

An effective way to achieve client satisfaction and avoid litigation is by using good communication techniques. The client should be consulted in all aspects of care. As you do this, demonstrate caring, empathy, and attentive listening. Incorporate the client's thoughts, feelings, and ideas into the plan of care.

## Cultural and Spiritual Considerations

### Cultural Considerations

As stated previously, holistic care includes identifying cultural and spiritual needs and concerns and formulating nursing diagnoses. As you write nursing diagnoses that relate to cultural needs, you should critically think of the appropriate long-term and short-term goals/outcomes that will be beneficial to your client. Let us now write corresponding goals for five nursing diagnoses that were listed in Chapter 3 for cultural needs. See Table 4–3.

### Spiritual Considerations

Let us now write corresponding goals/outcomes for the spiritual needs diagnoses that were listed in Chapter 3. See Table 4–4.

---

**TEST YOUR UNDERSTANDING**

Examine the following client scenario.

Mrs. Martinez is a 70-year-old Hispanic client who has had diabetes for 5 years. For 4 years her blood sugar was controlled on oral hypoglycemics. Six months ago she sustained a bruise on her great toe from wearing oversized shoes. This bruise became an open sore, which became infected "1 month ago." She used home remedies to treat the sore with no results.

She visited an outpatient clinic where her blood sugar was 400. She was admitted to the general hospital where her blood sugar was regulated on Insulin Humalin Regular and on an 1800-calorie ADA diet. She was taught insulin administration of Lente 30 units (the dose on which she was discharged). She was readmitted with a blood sugar of 500 and a history of extreme drowsiness. The wound that had shown signs of healing now had a bloody discharge.

During this interview she admitted not taking the insulin "because it is poisonous" and eating Mexican tortillas (her preference). She refused to eat the diet served in the hospital stating "I would rather die than eat what you serve. Why can't my sister bring my food? I want to get out of here so I can cook tortillas." She was found wandering in her room late that night, and stated "I am looking for the bathroom. I am never left in a room by myself." She cried out, "I have not seen my priest since you locked me in this place. I want him to be told everything about me."

**TABLE 4–3**

## Nursing Diagnoses and Corresponding Goals for Meeting Cultural Needs

| Nursing Diagnosis | Short-Term Goals | Long-Term Goals |
|---|---|---|
| 1. Noncompliance related to cultural beliefs | • Client will state his or her belief about the planned regimen of care.<br>• Client will discuss current plan being followed to solve the problem. | • Client will state the benefits of following the prescribed treatment. |
| 2. Knowledge deficit about the treatment regimen | • Client will verbalize concerns about the treatment plan. | • Client will verbalize adequate knowledge about the treatment plan. |
| 3. Risk for altered nutrition less than body requirements related to food idiosyncracies | • Client will verbalize a list of foods that is preferred. | • Client will select preferred food choices from a menu.<br>• Client will add items to the menu to show preference. |
| 4. Risk for injury related to unfamiliar environment | • Client will state concerns about new environment.<br>• Client will identify ways to prevent injury—and will be injury free. | • Client will remain injury free while in health-care setting. |
| 5. Powerlessness related to perceived inability to change current situations | • Client will verbalize inner feelings.<br>• Client will discuss past accomplishments: successes and failures. | • Client will engage in activities of daily living, within his or her limitations.<br>• Client will devise a plan to continue previous role within his or her limitations. |

**TABLE 4–4**

## Nursing Diagnosis and Corresponding Goals for Meeting Spiritual Needs

| Nursing Diagnosis | Short-Term Goals | Long-Term Goals |
|---|---|---|
| Spiritual Distress | • Client will verbalize his or her spiritual needs | • Client will verbalize satisfaction with his or her spiritual care. |

Write the goals that correspond with each nursing diagnosis.

| Clustered Data | Nursing Diagnosis | Short-Term Goals | Long-Term Goals |
|---|---|---|---|
| • Admits not taking insulin, "poisonous." <br> • Refuses to eat 1800-calorie diet. | Noncompliance | • Client will verbalize her beliefs about insulin. <br> • Client will discuss alternative measures being used to treat diabetes. <br> • Client will discuss relationship of diet to diabetes. <br> • Client will identify food idiosyncrasies on the first day of admission. | • Client will assist in devising a plan for meeting dietary needs both in the hospital and at home by the second day of hospitalization. <br> • Client will identify significant other who can be taught to assist in her care (insulin administration and diet planning). |
| • Treats open wound with home remedies <br> • Seeks health care mainly during a crisis. <br> • Thinks insulin is "poisonous." <br> • Wears oversized shoes. | Knowledge Deficit | • Client will discuss the following by the second day of admission: <br> —Infection and its causes <br> —Infection prevention <br> —Importance of keeping doctor's appointments <br> —Relationship of high blood sugar to infection on the feet | • Client will discuss diabetic foot care. <br> • Client will demonstrate proper foot care. <br> • Client will devise a plan for keeping appointments. <br> • Client will verbalize concerns about her care while at home between the second and third day of admission. |
| • Refuses to eat meal served in hospital. <br> • States "I would rather die than eat this food." | Risk for Altered Nutrition Less than Body Requirements | • Client will discuss food likes and dislikes. <br> • Client will assist in planning an 1800-calorie diet that includes her actual preferences on the first day of hospitalization. | • Client will discuss method of continuing this dietary regimen while at home before discharge. |

| Found wandering in room, stating "I am looking for the bathroom." | **Risk for Injury** | Client will discuss structural layout of room including call bell, light fixtures, and bathroom. | Client will identify significant other who can be companion while in hospital. |
| | | Client will state importance of calling for assistance when she needs to get out of bed and for other needs. | Client will be injury free throughout hospital stay. |
| | | Client will be injury free. | |
| States "I want to get out of here so I can cook my own food." | **Powerlessness** | Client will verbalize her need for autonomy between day one and two of hospitalization. | Client will discuss methods of her food preparation with dietician. |
| | | | Client will assist in making selection on menu and adding of preferential items between days two and three of hospitalization. |

## TEST YOUR UNDERSTANDING

Reread this critical thinking scenario from Chapter 3 that relates to nursing diagnoses. Refer to Figure 4–3 and use critical thinking to select the corresponding goals for each of these nursing diagnoses. Mark **T** for true for each goal (short-term and long-term) you consider to be correct.

   Mr. Jones, a 75-year-old male, is admitted to the unit with a medical diagnosis of "lumbar pain. This started 2 days ago." He has been in a wheelchair for 1 year after he suffered a stroke. He has had a Foley catheter in place for 3 months because of incontinence. His urinary output is less than 30 cc per hour and is concentrated. He is being fed through a gastrostomy tube. This has been in place for 6 months. He has one son who lives in Europe. He lost his wife 1 year ago. On admission his vital signs were: T—101, P—100, R—24. He wears a napkin, which shows no soiling on admission. He has lived in a nursing home for the last 6 months. You are asked to mark "T" for true only if all parts are accurately stated according to the client's condition.

| Nursing Diagnosis | Evidenced by | Related to | Short-Term Goals | Long-Term Goals |
|---|---|---|---|---|
| I  Acute pain | Complains of pain | Aging | • Client will rate pain on scale of one to ten, with ten as the greatest and one as the least.<br>• Client will describe nature of pain, for example, sharp, dull.<br>• Client will identify factors that relieve the pain.<br>• Client will identify pain as two or three at one to two hours after nursing interventions. | • Client will identify pain as one or two by the second day of hospitalization.<br>• Client will engage in activities of daily living. |
| II  Impaired mobility | Confinement to wheelchair | Stroke | • Client will describe the benefits of exercise: kegel, active, and passive.<br>• Client will return demonstration of the above exercises. | • Client will follow a planned schedule of exercise by at least day two of admission |
| III  Risk for infection | | Invasive procedure— Foley catheter | • Client will show an infection-free state evidenced by: temperature no greater than 98.6°F, pulse no greater than 80 beats per minute, urine clear and nonodorous. | • Client will show an infection-free state evidenced by: temperature no greater than 98.6°F, pulse no greater than 80 beats per minute, urine clear and nonodorous. |

FIGURE 4–3   Nursing diagnosis components with corresponding goals.

| IV | Altered elimination | Urine less than 30 cc per hour— concentrated | Immobility | • Urine will be amber within 4 hours of interventions. | • Client will eliminate 30–60 cc before the end of shift. |
|---|---|---|---|---|---|
| V | Possible social isolation | Needs more data | Altered family process— absent family member | • Client will discuss feelings about family and friends. | • Client will identify means of finding social comfort— probably contacting son, other family members, and friends. |
| VI | Possible grief— dysfunctional | Needs more data | Death of wife 1 year ago | • Client will verbalize feelings about loss of wife. | • Client will identify coping mechanisms according to verbalized need. |
| VII | Hyperthermia | T = 101 | Unknown etiology | • Client's temperature will be decreased within the next 4 hours. | • Client's temperature will be within the normal range of 98.6°F by the second hospital day. |
| VIII | Risk for constipation | | Immobility | • Client will identify foods high in roughage.<br>• Client will discuss the benefits in drinking 6 to 8 glasses of water daily. | • Client will have a soft formed bowel movement every 1 to 2 days while hospitalized.<br>• Client will identify regimen to follow after discharge. |
| IX | Risk for disuse syndrome | | Immobility | • Client will verbalize the benefits of exercise. | • Client will perform isotonic exercises at least twice daily. |

FIGURE 4–3    continued

## KEY TERMS

**cultural/spiritual**–Meeting specific needs of individual–holistic care.

**discharge goals**–Comprehensive benefits the client should derive while under your care and in the home setting.

**goals**–The benefit(s) the client should experience after the nursing intervention.

**legal/ethical considerations**–Goals that focus on awareness of client's rights, privileges, and safety.

**long-term goals**–More than can be expected on the first day, but while the client is still in your care. May be written in collaboration with staff–if so, specify.

**outcome criteria**–Used interchangeably with goals; that which is expected during and at the end of the planned therapy.

**priority/prioritize**–The clustering of patient data from most crucial (needs immediate attention) to least crucial (can be dealt with after the crucial problems are addressed). Goals are written to correspond with the nursing diagnoses prioritized list.

**recording**–The written account of the plan of care, individualized according to each client's need.

**sequencing**–All parts of the nursing process relate to each other–data, nursing diagnosis, goal, interventions, rationale evaluation (outcome criteria/goal).

**short-term goals**–Those that can be expected during your interaction with the client on the first day.

**standards of care**–Nursing care provided according to professional nursing standards designated by the American Nursing Association.

**teaching goals**–Those goals that relate to the nursing diagnosis "knowledge deficit."

## CHAPTER SUMMARY

In this chapter, the importance of relating each goal to its specific nursing diagnosis and individualizing to the client's needs was discussed. Short-term goals were differentiated from long-term ones. The relevance of nursing interventions to professional nursing standards was emphasized. Planning was presented as a comprehensive approach to client care, which should always include cultural and spiritual concerns and ethical and legal issues.

## NURSING CHECKLIST

- Prerequisites for writing goals:
  - —Be specific about the one nursing diagnosis for which the goal is written and show correlation.
  - —Write short-term and long-term goals for each nursing diagnosis.
- Goals must be client-centered (not nurse-centered), must be realistic (can be attained by the client), must be measurable (see measurable terminology in the appendix on Delmar's Web site), must designate a time frame within which they are to be realized.
- Discharge goals—These should be compiled inclusive of all care given to clients and should be discussed throughout the client's encounter with the nurse. They should be rehearsed with the client at the time of discharge.
- Teaching goals—These should address the knowledge base of all clients.
- Cultural goals—Should deal with specific differences of clients.
- Spiritual goals—Address spiritual needs of clients.
- Ethical goals—Prevent legal client/staff encounters.
- Planning nursing interventions—The actions the nurse plans to take to address each client problem should be outlined and labeled as: independent, dependent, and collaborative.
- Recording—Document all nursing care plans legibly and comprehensively to facilitate continuity of care, collaborate, and avoid duplication.
- SOAPI charting/SOAPIER charting—Deals with:
  - —Subjective—what the client says
  - —Objective—what the nurse sees in relationship to the subjective
  - —Assessment—what the nurse finds (physical assessment)
  - —Plan—goals—short and long term
  - —Intervention—actions the nurse takes to address the client's problem/diagnosis (independent, dependent, collaborative)
  - —Evaluation—determine if the goals are realized (goals met, goals not met)
  - —Revision—if the goals are not met, rework the plan through all the stages: data collection to evaluation.
- Standards of care—All client goals must adhere to the ANA professional standards of care.

## REVIEW QUESTIONS

Select the one best answer.

1. The planning phase
   a. follows the nursing diagnosis formulation.
   b. follows evaluation.
   c. focuses only on the interview.
   d. ends with auscultation.

2. Prioritizing means
   a. accepting all subjective data as fact.
   b. dealing with the most critical problem first.
   c. recording all data before leaving the unit.
   d. following the instructor's suggestions without question.

3. Which of the following describes a short-term goal?
   a. Written sentences are short and precise.
   b. They are more easily achieved.
   c. Achievement is generally expected within an 8-hour encounter with the client.
   d. They are truly the discharge goals.

4. Which best describes a well-written goal? It is
   a. nurse-centered and easily evaluated.
   b. clear and concise and has time constraints.
   c. prioritized and realistic.
   d. client-centered, has time constraints, and is realistic.

5. What characterizes a long-term goal? A long-term goal
   a. is a result of their inability to show positive results.
   b. generally requires more than a 24-hour period to be realized.
   c. generally requires at least 6 months to be realized.
   d. is more difficult to formulate than short-term goals.

6. Teaching goals for clients refer to
   a. medication errors.          c. insulin administration.
   b. late charting.              d. knowledge deficit.

7. Discharge goals are best addressed
   a. from the day of admission.        c. on the third day of admission.
   b. when the client asks about them.  d. at the time of discharge.

8. Which of the following best describes nursing interventions? Nursing interventions are
   a. actions that facilitate goal realization.
   b. actions that facilitate good interview techniques.
   c. actions that guide the nursing diagnosis.
   d. unmet goals.

9. What are benefits of proper documentation? Proper documentation
   a. lists all concerns voiced by clients.
   b. follows a concise way of charting all physical and psychological problems.
   c. prevents repetition and facilitates collaboration.
   d. prevents misrepresentation by nursing personnel.

10. The "A" in SOAPIER stands for
    a. what the client says.      c. what the nurse finds.
    b. what the nurse sees.       d. what the physician writes.

11. Standards that guide nursing interventions are set by
    a. World Health Organization (WHO).
    b. American Nurses Association (ANA).
    c. American Red Cross (ARC).
    d. Oncology Nursing Organization (ONC).

12. ANA standards protect the
    a. nurse's rights to practice.      c. patient's rights to care.
    b. teacher's rights to instruct.    d. doctor's rights to practice.

13. Goals that include physiological, psychological, legal, ethical, cultural, and spiritual concerns can best be described as
    a. long term.                  c. holistic.
    b. "good" outcome criteria.    d. baseline data.

## ANSWERS TO CASE STUDIES

Prioritizing (page 99) The correct order of the diagnoses from most pressing to least crucial is paragraph 1, Ineffective breathing pattern; paragraph 3, Pain related to trauma of surgery; paragraph 2, Ineffective airway clearance; paragraph 5, Nutrition more than body requirements; paragraph 6, Risk for altered skin integrity; and paragraph 4, Constipation.

Test Your Understanding (page 120) All short-term and long-term goals should be marked with a T for true.

**Client's Initial RB**
**Room # 459**

**Age 65**

**Nursing Care Plan**
**Medical Diagnosis: Chronic Obstructive Pulmonary Disease (COPD)**

| Ordered & Selected Data | Nursing Diagnosis | Goals | Interventions | Rationale Evaluation |
|---|---|---|---|---|
| Subjective: Client states "I can't breathe." | Altered breathing pattern related to altered lung ventilation and evidenced by restlessness & respirations of 45 beats per minute | Short term: Client will demonstrate improved breathing 28–30 respirations within 1 hour. Color will be less ashed (pale pink). | Independent Nursing Functions: • Continue to nurse in high Fowler's position. • Reassure client that everything is being done to improve condition. • Stay with patient. • Adjust O₂ as needed. | Provides comfort Facilitates breathing Develops trust Decreases anxiety |
| Objective: Color ashen | | | | |
| T 100.2 P 110 R 45 BP 160/100 | | Long term: Client's breathing will decrease to 20–25 beats per minute within 6 hours. | • Apply cool cloth to forehead. • Monitor VS q15 minutes • Report condition as necessary. Dependent Give medications as ordered. Administer IV fluids as ordered. Implement new orders. Collaborative Discuss O₂ therapy with therapist as necessary. Provide expert input into this aspect of care. | Decreases temperature Provides for reassessment Medications & IV fluids are generally prescribed to improve the client's condition and prevent or improve dehydration. |
| Lying in high Fowler's position restless—O₂ via nasal cannula at 3 liters per minute | | | | |
| Lung fields reveal: Crackles & rales in lower bases bilaterally Hemoglobin—10 g/dh Hematocrit—31 | Ineffective airway clearance related to nonproductive cough—tenacious sputum & generalized weakness & inability to cough effectively | Crackles & rhonchal will be less audible within 6 hours. | Independent • Increase fluid intake: 800 cc 0700–1500 500 cc 1500–2300 200 cc 2300–0700 Encourage use of inspirometer q 1 to 2 hours. Encourage coughing & deep breathing every 2 hours. | Loosens secretion from respiratory tract Promotes alveolar gas exchange Reference: Phipps et al., *Medical surgical nursing* (4th ed.). |

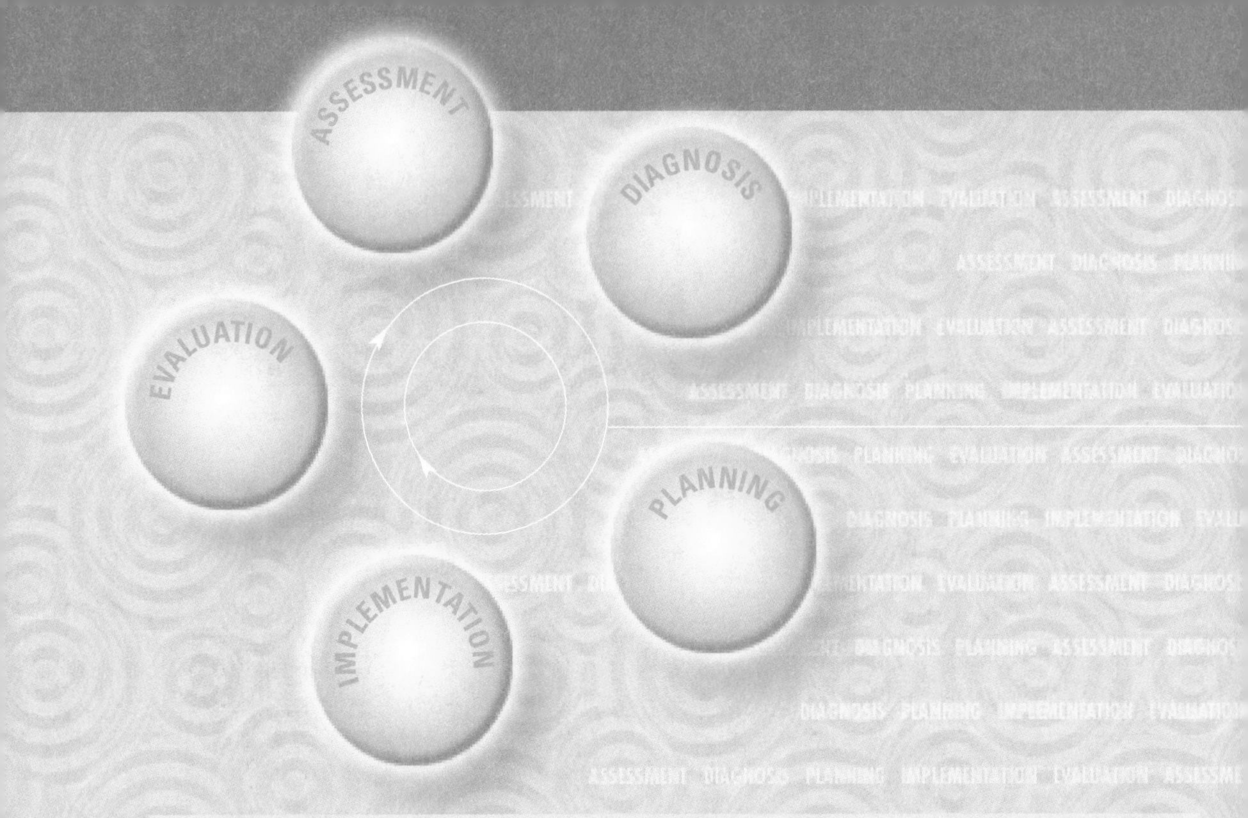
ASSESSMENT
DIAGNOSIS
PLANNING
IMPLEMENTATION
EVALUATION

## CHAPTER OUTLINE

# Implementation

## Objectives

Upon completion of this chapter, you should be able to:

- Define implementation.
- Determine the importance of verbal reports.
- Utilize information from a verbal report to examine previously written nursing interventions.
- Determine if the need for the intervention still exists.
- Determine the rationale for each nursing intervention.
- Identify equipment and supplies necessary to safely carry out the nursing interventions.
- Share the underlying principles for each intervention with the client as you perform the nursing procedures.
- Share client's response to nursing interventions through verbal reports.
- Utilize various methods of charting to record client's response to nursing interventions.
- Discuss the legal aspects of charting.
- Discuss standardized graphic and assessment flow sheets and their use in documentation.

## KEY TERMS

| | | |
|---|---|---|
| client's response | flow sheet | underlying principle |
| client's status | legal aspect | verbal report |
| critical pathway | rationale | |
| existing need | recording | |

Implementation is the actual carrying out of the nursing interventions. In the planning phase you wrote the nursing interventions to correlate with each goal. In this phase you put them into action and include the rationale for each action. The significance of the verbal report will also be determined. Various forms of documentation are assessed and legal implications are discussed.

## VERBAL REPORT

The **verbal report** has great significance in that it enables you to get current information about the client. It helps you to determine whether your nursing interventions should be implemented as previously written or if new ones should be added.

### Identifying the Client's Status from the Verbal Report

Remember that the **client's status** may change from minute to minute. Remember also that many people may be involved in the care of the same client. Nurses also work various shifts around the clock. It is therefore crucial that a report of the client's current status be passed on to the next caregiver so an intelligent assessment of the client can be made. This report is best given orally from one nurse to another. It is very important that you take an accurate report from the person who is sharing the information.

Points to remember when taking the report:

- Meet in a well-lit area.
  Rationale: Provides for good note-taking, also enables you to determine nonverbal communication from the reporter.
- Bring pad and pen for jotting down notes.
  Rationale: Record significant times and events to assure they are not forgotten.

- Listen attentively to all information shared. Wait until the reporter has finished discussing your client. Then ask for missing information and for clarification of points that are unclear.
  Rationale: Helps you to fully assess your client's status and needs and to determine existing need for specific interventions.
- Review your nursing interventions and determine those that should still be implemented.
  Rationale: Provides for critical thinking and correct decision making.
- Rearrange the needed interventions according to priority.
  Rationale: Provides for efficiency in nursing care; that means that the client's most pressing needs are met first.

## Determining Existing Need for Specific Interventions

The report you receive may be called the change of shift report. This may be given by the nurse who works the 2300 to 0700 shift. If you are working the 0700 to 1500 shift, bear in mind that the nurse from whom you received your report also had received the report from another nurse on the previous shift. That means many changes could have occurred in the client's condition since you wrote your nursing interventions. The client's condition could have improved or worsened. A transfer to another room could have occurred. For these reasons, you need to examine your interventions carefully to determine those that are necessary and should still be implemented. You should identify the **existing need** for new interventions.

## Determining the Rationale for Each Nursing Intervention

The **rationale** is the scientific reason for choosing a specific action for a stated nursing intervention. It is most often based on tested theory and should therefore be expected to produce a specific outcome (goal). Use a good nursing reference and correlate the corresponding rationale with the nursing intervention. Because the rationale explains the reason for a specific nursing intervention, it will help you understand the **underlying principle**, which is the reason for an action and the benefit to be derived by the client.

Refer to the following Nursing in Action Case Study to refresh your understanding of the process by which the nurse develops interventions for the client.

## Case Study—Mrs. Martinez

Mrs. Martinez is a 70-year-old Hispanic client who has had diabetes for 5 years. For 4 years her blood sugar was controlled on oral hypoglycemics. Six months ago she sustained a bruise on her great toe from wearing oversized shoes. This bruise became an open sore, which became infected "1 month ago." She used home remedies to treat the sore with no results. She visited an outpatient clinic where her blood sugar was 400.

She was admitted to the general hospital where her blood sugar was regulated on Insulin Humalin Regular and on an 1800-calorie ADA diet. She was taught insulin administration of 70/30 units (the dose on which she was discharged). She was readmitted with a blood sugar of 500 and a history of extreme drowsiness. The wound that had shown signs of healing now had a bloody discharge. During this interview she admitted not taking the insulin "because it is poisonous" and eating Mexican tortillas (her preference). She refused to eat the diet served in the hospital stating, "I would rather die than eat what you serve. Why can't my sister bring my food? I want to get out of here so I can cook tortillas." She was found wandering in her room late that night, and stated, "I am looking for the bathroom. I am never left in a room by myself." She cried out, "I have not seen my priest since you locked me in this place. I want him to be told everything about me."

Refer to the Nursing Care Plan for Mrs. Martinez.

## Implementing the Identified Nursing Interventions

The following steps are critical to successful implementation.

1. Identifying equipment and supplies necessary to safely carry out the nursing interventions
   Observe the following points:
   - Be sure to gather all necessary supplies prior to starting your intervention.
   - Always check to be sure they are in working order. If the type of equipment is specified in a written order, be sure they are chosen according to the order; remember that equipment is generally age-specific and should therefore be chosen for the right age group.
   - Take all equipment to the area of treatment before beginning.
2. Sharing the underlying principles with the client
   Tell the client what you are about to do and ensure privacy before beginning. These actions will accomplish the following:
   - Reduce fear and prevent invasion of privacy from others.
   - Provide information about the care provided.

**Nursing Care Plan**
**Care Plan for Mrs. Martinez**

| Clustered Data | Nursing Diagnosis | Short-Term Goals | Long-Term Goals | Nursing Interventions |
|---|---|---|---|---|
| Subjective:<br>• Admitted not taking insulin, "poisonous"<br>Objective:<br>• Refused to eat 1800-calorie diet | **Noncompliance** | • Client will verbalize her beliefs about insulin.<br>• Client will discuss alternative measures being used to treat diabetes.<br>• Client will discuss relationship of diet to diabetes.<br>• Client will identify food idiosyncrasies on the first day of admission. | • Client will assist in devising a plan for meeting dietary needs both in the hospital and at home by the second day of hospitalization.<br>• Client will identify significant other who can be taught to assist in her care (insulin administration and diet planning). | • Ask client to tell what she knows about insulin. (Provide atmosphere conducive to development of trust/effective communication—listening, open-ended questions, privacy, and empathy.)<br>• Ask client to name substances she uses to treat diabetes.<br>• Tell client that her body, which used to secrete insulin necessary to break down carbohydrates and sugars, is no longer working but the insulin injections will help the body to do similar things and she will be able to control her blood sugar if she eats a diet as close as possible to what her doctor orders.<br>• Help client to select food exchanges that closely correlate with Mexican food and with the prescribed diet.<br>• Ask client to name significant other who can assist in insulin administration and meal planning and cooking. |
| Subjective:<br>• Treats open wound with home remedies<br>• Seeks health care mainly during a crisis<br>• Thinks insulin is "poisonous"<br>Objective:<br>• Wears oversized shoes | **Knowledge Deficit** | • Client will discuss the following by the second day of admission:<br>—Infection and its causes<br>—Infection prevention<br>—Importance of keeping doctor's appointments<br>—Relationship of high blood sugar to infection on the feet<br>—Problems related to wearing oversized shoes | • Client will discuss diabetic foot care.<br>• Client will demonstrate proper foot care.<br>• Client will devise a plan for keeping appointments.<br>• Client will verbalize concerns about her care while at home between the second and third day of admission. | • Make a chart to describe the infectious process and show client redness/discoloration of skin.<br>• Discuss pain.<br>• Discuss proper foot washing, drying, and inspection, wearing proper fitting shoes, and reporting of any problems with feet to doctor right away.<br>• Teach client that when the skin breaks, organisms enter that cause infection, which is easier to get when the blood sugar is high. |

*continues*

**Nursing Care Plan (continued)**

| Clustered Data | Nursing Diagnosis | Short-Term Goals | Long-Term Goals | Nursing Interventions |
|---|---|---|---|---|
| | | | | • Teach client that blood sugar problems can be prevented by keeping doctor's appointments. |
| Objective: <br> • Refused to eat meal served in hospital <br> Subjective: <br> • States "I would rather die than eat this food" | **Risk for Altered Nutrition Less than Body Requirements** | • Client will discuss food likes and dislikes. <br> • Client will assist in planning an 1800-calorie diet that includes her actual preferences on the first day of hospitalization. | • Client will discuss method of continuing this dietary regimen while at home before discharge. | • Discuss the allowable items on an 1800-calorie ADA diet. <br> • Assist client to choose food exchanges from Mexican foods. |
| Objective: <br> • Found wandering in room, stating, <br> Subjective: <br> • "I am looking for the bathroom." | **Risk for Injury** | • Client will discuss structural layout of room including call bell, light fixtures, and bathroom. <br> • Client will state importance of calling for assistance when she needs to get out of bed and for other needs. <br> • Client will be injury free. | • Client will identify significant other who can be companion while in hospital. <br> • Client will be injury free throughout hospital stay. | • Orient client to bed and its operation (pillows, side rails, etc.). <br> • Have client operate call bell and light. <br> • Instruct on importance of calling for assistance when needed especially when there is need to get out of bed. <br> • Leave room free of clutter at all times. <br> • Identify individual who can stay with client especially during the night. |
| • States "I want to get out of here so I can cook my own food." | **Powerlessness** | • Client will verbalize her need for autonomy between day one and two of hospitalization. | • Client will discuss methods of her food preparation with dietician. <br> • Client will assist in making selection on menu and adding of preferential items between days two and three of hospitalization. | • Have client talk about hospitalization care, diet, insulin, and all her concerns. <br> • Have client assist in making selection on menu. |

134

- Develop a trusting relationship between the client and the nurse.
- Facilitate communication.
- Meet the client's teaching needs.

Be sure to explain the procedure before beginning and continue the explanation throughout the process. This should be done at the client's level of understanding.

3. Sharing client's response to nursing interventions through verbal reports

Verbal reporting is an integral part of the nursing intervention. It serves to communicate to the health-care team:

- The **client's response** (or outcome of the nursing interventions)
- New observations—physical and/or psychological
- Need for change in a treatment schedule
- Problems that need instant collaboration
- Problems that can be deferred
- Interchange of ideas among team members
- Decisions made
- Critical thinking strategies used
- Provides for efficient problem solving among many people
- Confidence expressed to the students by the client
- Questions asked and points clarified

The verbal report also serves as an avenue for constructive criticism and provides for face-to-face contact. This reveals feelings and emotions that often convey the need for delayed or quick action.

## METHODS OF RECORDING THE NURSING INTERVENTIONS AND THEIR OUTCOMES

Nursing is a profession where **recording** or documentation is of paramount importance. It is the cornerstone of proving or disproving legal issues. Remember to document the interventions and their outcomes. There are various methods of documentation/recording, including:

- Narrative
- SOAP
- SOAPIE
- Focus DAR

- PIE charting
- Charting by exception
- Critical pathways
- Computerized

Let us now learn about each method of documentation/recording and examine some examples.

## Narrative Charting

Narrative charting requires documentation of all activities surrounding the care provided and the client's response to the procedures. The date and time of each action is recorded and events are written sequentially. That is, they should be written at the time of implementation. This means notes are written as soon as possible after implementation. In these notes you also record your assessment findings prior to, during, and after your implementation. The disadvantages of narrative notes include: they are longer, less concise, and invite the reader to search through paragraphs to find specific problems. To address this problem, some health-care facilities use supporting charts for charting routine situations such as diet and vital signs. These charts are often called flow charts. Let's examine this narrative charting.

**EXAMPLE:**    Narrative Charting

5/16/20xx, 0730 Mrs. R.M. lying in bed in semi-Fowler's position. Color pink, skin warm and dry; oriented to time place and person. Foley catheter in situ with 200 cc concentrated urine in Foley bag. Lungs clear bilaterally; no neurological deficits detected in lower extremity (responds to painful stimuli, toes warm to touch, denies numbness and tingling, capillary refill less than 3 seconds, all pulses palpable). Dressing at site of abdominal incision wet with moderate to large amount of serosanguineous drainage. Jackson Pratt drainage system out of wound (found in bed clothes).

0745 Abdominal dressing changed according to physician's order. Client teaching regarding care of tube site done; client reassured of intactness of incision site and need to replace drainage tube.

0800 Assisted Dr. Black with reinsertion of corrugated drainage tube. *Patricia Henry, University of Mohawk, student nurse* (Patricia Henry, UMSN).

## SOAP Notes

The SOAP format uses an interdisciplinary approach. The client's problems are identified and listed. Each member of the team then charts relevant information about each problem.

The acronym is defined as:

S–Subjective data: That which the client states. These data should be in quotation marks. If the client does not verbalize anything relevant to the problem, then "None" is recorded.

O–Objective data: Includes the visible signs and symptoms as they relate to the problem and the laboratory and diagnostic tests and their results.

A–Assessment: In-depth assessment is done to determine the cause and effect of related and underlying factors.

P–Plan: The steps to be taken to address the client's problems.

## SOAPIE

Another form of charting takes the SOAP format further by including "I" and "E." The SOAP portion is the same as described previously. The additional letters mean:

I–Interventions: These are the nursing orders that will be implemented on the client's behalf.

E–Evaluation: Determines if the interventions successfully dealt with the client's problems.

- Advantages of SOAP and SOAPIE documentation:
  1. Problems can be quickly identified from a prepared list.
  2. All members of the team become cognizant of the problems. They share in the interventions, implementation, and evaluation of outcomes.
  3. Team collaboration determines problem resolution and new strategy development.

- Disadvantage

  The concise approach to documentation with these formats may cause nurses to feel restricted in the information they want to share as opposed to narrative charting.

EXAMPLE:    SOAPIE Documentation

S–"I cannot eat. I feel bloated."
O–Abdomen distended but soft.

A—Third day postoperation: Passing flatus but only occasionally. Bowel sounds hypoactive in all four quadrants. No bowel movement since surgery.

P—Client will evacuate bowel of feces within next 2 hours on 5/20/20xx.

I—Hold breakfast. Administer Fleet® enema according to physician's standing order for third postoperative day.

E—Client had medium-sized bowel movement, soft and formed. Stated "I am feeling less bloated."

You should be aware that the problem list is generally developed when the client is first admitted. New problems are added as they occur; old problems are deleted as they are resolved. The date and time for these occurrences should be documented. Problems that the nurse identifies are written after the format of the NANDA Nursing Diagnoses list and may include actual and potential problems.

## Focus DAR Charting

With focus DAR charting, information is organized around the acronym DAR.

D—Stands for data, which includes the subjective statement and objective observations that created the need for the documentation.

A—Stands for action; interventions are documented in this section.

R—Stands for response; results of the treatment are recorded here.

This method of charting is not restricted to identified problems, but may include wellness aspects such as health promotion, disease prevention, client teaching, and client accomplishments. It may also include identified nursing diagnoses.

EXAMPLE:   Focus DAR Charting

| DATE | TIME | FOCUS | NOTE |
|------|------|-------|------|
| 9/30/20xx | 10:00 A.M. | Dressing Changed | Data: <br> • Client to be discharged on 10/1/20xx <br> • Requires daily dressing. <br> • No previous instruction on this procedure. <br> • Client verbalizes desire to learn. |

| | | | | Action: • Discuss methods of transmitting organisms to wound. • Share the positive outcome of not contaminating wound. • Demonstrate good hand-washing technique. • Demonstrate donning the gloves. • Demonstrate the procedure for removing soiled dressing and replacing sterile dressing. Response: • After teaching session client was able to answer 95% of questions regarding bacteria transmission and benefits of avoiding contamination of wound. • Donned gloves without difficulty. • Removed soiled dressing and replaced sterile dressing with minimal coaching. |
| 10/1/20xx | 10:00 A.M. | Dressing Changed | | Client performed all steps without coaching. Expressed confidence in procedure. "Relatives will come to hospital to take her home after lunch." |

## PIE Charting

The elements of the acronym are defined as:

P–Problem
I–Intervention
E–Evaluation

PIE charting is nurse-centered. The nursing diagnoses are the identified problems. This format is considered narrow in scope because it does not use the multidisciplinary approach. Also, there is no selected listing of nursing diagnoses at the time of the admission assessment. It is easy to use because it mainly states the problem, identifies what is to be done about it, and evaluates the outcome. There are times, however, when an A and D are added to form ADPIE. The charting then includes A for assessment and D for diagnosis. Every 24 hours all problems are reviewed to determine resolution of client's problems and the need to add new ones to the list. This prevents duplication and confirms the client's current health status.

EXAMPLE: PIE Charting (Refers to previous Case Study for Mrs. Martinez)

| DATE | PROBLEM | NURSING DIAGNOSIS |
|---|---|---|
| 8/30/20xx | #1 | Noncompliance regarding diabetes management. Failure to:<br>1. adhere to 1800 calories, ADA diet.<br>2. take insulin—30 units 70/30 daily.<br>3. observe foot care regimen. |
| | Intervention for Problem #1 | **P(#1)** Assess client's cognitive and educational level.<br>**P(#1)** Determine client's knowledge base about: diabetes, insulin therapy, and self-care to include care of the feet.<br>**P(#1)** Determine client's readiness to learn including (a) self-perception, (b) roll relationships, and (c) coping (stress tolerance).<br>**P(#1)** Instruct client on the benefits of (1) eating prescribed diet (identify food idiosyncrasies and discuss exchange), (2) taking insulin as prescribed, (3) care of the feet.<br>**P(#1)** Involve significant other and other caring individuals in the home-care regimen. Provide instruction in Spanish. Use diagrammatic illustrations. |
| | Evaluation for Problem #1 | Client reads at grade 4 level. Prior instructions given in English. (Nurse does not speak Spanish. Literature supplied in Spanish but nurse unable to clearly explain.)<br>Client's son-in-law is bilingual. Admitted understanding information in last teaching session; expressed willingness to help client follow regimen. |

## Charting by Exception

Charting by exception means that only developments beyond the norms are documented. These norms or standards are developed by individual hospitals, and nurses are instructed in their use to determine the client's status. If changes occur in client status (outside of the recorded norm), thorough documentation of the changes occurs. In this case any of the charting formats may be used for documentation. Nurses are expected to make check marks on forms (flow sheets) to show that the client's condition remains within the acceptable norm.

- Advantages of charting by exception:
  1. Time efficient
  2. Changes in client status readily detectable
- Disadvantages of charting by exception:
  1. Longer period of time required for personnel education regarding chart forms
  2. Difficult for personnel on next shift to follow specific changes

## Critical Pathways

**Critical pathways** are guidelines that outline specific expectations for a client's recovery on a day-by-day basis. These guidelines contain written goals and interventions. They vary according to the medical diagnosis and/or the surgical intervention. The nurse is responsible for making a check mark against the goals and the interventions as they are carried out and met. If the client's recovery does not follow the daily expectations, there should be detailed documentation describing the variation. See an example of a critical pathway on page 147.

## Computerized Charting

In today's health-care environment, computerized charting is the norm more than the exception. The many benefits to this documentation format include:

- Easy accessibility of information
- Time and space efficient
- Accurate information
- Facilitates sharing of information across disciplines
- Generates specific patient data such as laboratory profiles and times and dates of medications administered

- Generates individualized data sheets for inputting of concise and accurate information
- Encourages accuracy of performance by the nurse because names and actions of all users are documented

## LEGAL ASPECTS OF CHARTING AND IMPLICATIONS FOR ACCURATE CHARTING

The **legal aspects** of charting mean that whatever is written or not written in the client's chart has legal implications. Careful thought should be given to all entries to protect the client, the nurse, and the health-care institution from legal action. Table 5–1 lists principles that will promote good charting technique.

### TABLE 5–1
### Charting Principles

| PRINCIPLES | ACTION | RATIONALE |
|---|---|---|
| 1. Do not erase. | Draw a line through the wrong entry, sign your name and enter the correct information. | May convey an attempt at cover-up information. |
| 2. Include the date and time. | Chart sequentially and give the date and time of each entry. | Reveals the sequence in which events occurred. |
| 3. Do not leave spaces between lines of entry. | Endeavor to fill the total space on each line or draw lines to fill empty spaces. | Protects from erroneous entry by others. |
| 4. Be factual. | Write the facts as you observe them including quotations from the client. | Avoids subjectivity and bias. |
| 5. Avoid criticism of client and health-care workers. | Chart objectively and avoid critical statements and name calling. For example: Do not say "Nurse M. Lewis took 2 hours to take the client's BP after she was informed that it was 90/50. Subsequently the client slipped into a coma." | Statements have implications. Subjective statements convey unprofessional behavior and poor judgment. |

*continues*

## TABLE 5-1  Continued

### Charting Principles

| PRINCIPLES | ACTION | RATIONALE |
|---|---|---|
| 6. Clarify all unclear orders. | Ask questions about illegible and possible wrong orders such as names and dosage of medications. | The nurse is as liable as the physician for carrying out a wrong order. |

## FLOW SHEETS

**Flow sheets** are simplified chart forms that allow for placing a simple check mark against client care procedures and observations carried out by the nurse.

The advantages of flow sheets:

- Information is readily available.
- Time efficient—requires a check mark instead of paragraphs of documentation.
- Avoids duplication.
- Saves space, less bulky.
- Comprehensive enough to include client goals, interventions, and dates and times of activities.

Points to remember:

- The flow sheet is filled out completely or tasks cannot be verified as completed.
- Be sure to use age-specific, unit-specific, and information-specific flow sheets for your clients. Some flow sheets are for adults, some for pediatric clients, and others pertain only to high-risk areas such as critical care units.
- A check mark does not convey major changes in a client's condition. Detailed charting in another documentation format is required to describe events—such as assessment, interventions, and outcomes—when these changes occur in your client.
- Sign your name on the flow sheet in the space provided.

See example of a pediatric flow sheet on page 144.
See example of discharge flow sheet on page 146.

## Pediatric Flow Sheet Child 2 to 10 Years Old

Name _____

Nickname_____    Sex _____

Address_____    Name of Parents: First _____    Last _____

Occupation of Parents _____

Daytime Telephone _____

Daytime Address _____

Street                     City                      State                     Zip

Source of History _____

Chief Complaint _____    Time of Onset _____

    Location _____

    Individuals Involved_____    Teacher _____    Parents _____

    Duration _____    Aggravated Factors _____    Relieving Factors _____

Childhood Diseases   Measles ____   Mumps ____   Rubella ____   Chicken Pox ____   Whooping Cough ____

Previous Screening Tests   Results _____    Dates _____

Environmental Hazards   School _____    Home _____

Sleep Patterns _____

Diet   24-Hour Diet Recall _____    Likes/Dislikes _____

Current Medications   Prescription _____    Over the Counter _____

    Tobacco Use _____

    Alcohol          _____

    Drugs            _____

Day in the Life of the Child _____

Religious Affiliation _____

Mental Status:  Oriented to Time _____    Place _____    Person _____

Language Skills _____    Number Skills _____

Motor Skills _____    Ties Shoelaces    Yes _____    No _____

    Buttons Shirt    Yes _____    No _____

    Uses Scissors   Yes _____    No _____

    Discriminates from Right to Left    Yes _____    No _____


Past Medical History

Hospitalizations _____

Illnesses _____

Growth Retardation _____    Social _____    Physiological _____

Review of systems _____

Current Weight   _____

Weight Loss        _____

Weight Gain        _____

Skin   Erythema _____    Lesions _____    Ecchymosis _____    Rash _____    Itching _____

    Sores _____    Dryness _____


Head

Headache _____    Circumference _____Shape _____    Symmetry _____    Mobility _____    Control _____

    Head Injury _____

Eyes   Vision _____    Pain _____    Redness _____    Excessive Tearing _____

Double Vision _____


Ears

Hearing _____    Tinnitus _____    Vertigo _____    Ear Ache _____    Infection _____

Nose and Sinuses
Frequent Colds _____   Itching _____   Discharge _____   Stuffiness _____   Nosebleeds _____
Allergies _____   Hay Fever _____ .

Mouth and Throat
Teeth  Caries _____   Missing _____   Gums Bleeding _____Swollen Tongue _____   Tongue Coated _____
Tonsils Swollen _____   Throat Sore _____   Hoarseness _____   Last Dental Exam _____

Neck
Lymph Nodes Palpable _____   Stiffness _____

Breasts
Abnormal Growth _____   Discharge from Nipples _____   Pain _____   Tenderness _____

Respiratory
Cough _____   Productive _____   Nonproductive _____   Color of Sputum _____
Wheezing _____   Hemoptysis _____   Tuberculosis_____   Asthma_____   Bronchitis _____
Pertusis _____   Pneumonia _____   Last Chest X-Ray _____

Cardiac
Congenital Problems _____   Rheumatic Fever _____   Dyspnea _____   Orthopnea _____
Chest Pain _____   Palpitation _____   Edema _____   Paroxysmal Nocturnal Dyspnea _____
Heart Murmur _____

Gastrointestinal
Distended Abdomen _____   Vomiting _____   Diarrhea _____   Blood in Vomit _____
Blood in Stool _____   Color of Stool _____   Color of Vomit _____   Abdominal Pain _____

Urinary
Nocturnal Enuresis _____   Polyurea _____   Burning on Micturition _____   Pain on Micturition _____
Hesitancy _____   Infections _____

Genitalia Male
Hypospadias _____   Hyperspadias _____   Penile Discharge _____   Undescended Testicle _____
Testicular Pain _____   Circumcision _____   Penile Sores _____   Sexual Abuse _____

Genitalia Female
Vaginal Discharge _____   Sores on Labia _____   Malformation _____   Sexual Abuse _____
Itching _____   Menstruation _____   Dysmenorrhea _____   Menorrhagia _____   Date of Menarche _____

Musculoskeletal
Muscle Stiffness _____   Muscle Pain _____   Joint Stiffness _____   Joint Pain _____
Joint Swelling _____   Muscle Weakness _____   Immobility _____
Joint Weakness _____   Activity Intolerance _____

Neurological
Seizures _____   IQ _____   Fainting _____   Numbness _____   Tingling _____
Weakness _____   Tremors _____

Endocrine
Heat and Cold Intolerance _____   Polyurea _____   Juvenile Diabetes _____

Blood Profile
Increased WBC _____   Decreased WBC _____   Anemia _____   Hematocrit _____
Hemoglobin _____   Easy Bruising _____   Bleeding in Joints _____

Source: Bates, B. (2002). *A guide to physical examination and history taking.* Philadelphia: Lippincott.

**Discharge Flow Sheet—Begins on Day of Admission**

Personal Information:  Age_____  Sex_____  Weight_____  Height_____  Religion_____  Dietary Restriction_____
Admission Date: _____
Admission Diagnosis: _____
Client Signature: _____  Nurse's Signature: _____

| | Potential Nursing Diagnoses | Goals | Interventions | Yes | No |
|---|---|---|---|---|---|
| Day 1 | (Admission) Risk for high anxiety state related to unknown factors: • new environment • diagnostic tests • surgical preparation | Client will achieve moderate to mild anxiety state after: Orientation to hospital environment Explanation of laboratory and diagnostic tests Presurgery preparation | Client teaching: Orient to room: • call bell • high-low bed • over bed table • bathroom • night light • visiting hours • surgical preparation NPO state • surgery schedule • consent form | | |
| Day 2 | (Post Op day 1) Self-care deficit Pain | Will perform activities of daily living within limitations Will rate pain as 2 to 3 on scale of 1 to 10 | Client teaching: Coughing and deep breathing Use of incentive inspirometer Oxygen administration Intravenous maintenance Bathing, feeding, voiding Positioning, pain control | | |
| Day 3 | (Post Op day 2) Activity intolerance risk for infection | Will be injury free (no falls) Will maintain infection-free state (wound healing by first intention) | Client teaching: Proper body mechanics Use of assistive devices (walker, cane, as ordered) Wound care (in hospital and at home) | | |
| Day 4 day of discharge | (Post Op day 3) Knowledge deficit (self-care management) | Knowledge deficit related to: Medications, home hazards, caregiver roles, self-care activities, other home care assistance, financial resources | Client teaching: Medication (frequency dose, time of administration) Home hazards (throw rugs, stairs, walker) Hygiene, wound care, diet, water intake Caregiver role (assistance with hygiene medication and daily activities) Financial assistance (social worker) | | |

146

## Example of Critical Pathway for a Client Admitted for Lumbar Laminectomy

Scenario: Mrs. Donna Allen is a 55-year-old female who was admitted to the hospital with complaints of low back pain over a period of 6 months. She states the pain is severe, has become worse month by month, and is now continuous and is radiating down her legs. A computerized axial tomography (CAT) scan revealed degeneration of lumbar 4 and 5. She is diagnosed with herniated nucleus pulposus. She is scheduled for laminectomy the next day at 1300.

Refer to the following information: assessment, nursing diagnoses, goals/interventions, and discharge teaching (pp. 147–150).

**Preoperative Assessment**

Date              Time

**Allergy:** Penicillin
**Mental Status:** Alert oriented to time, place, and person.
**Elimination:** No problems with voiding. Has at least one bowel movement a day.
**Neurological:** Radiating pain to both legs "pins and needles." Pulses palpable 2+, extremities warm to touch.

**Diet/Nutrition:**  Height:          5 feet, 3 inches
                    Weight:          250 pounds
                    Body Frame:      medium, ideal body weight 127 pounds
                                     123 pounds overweight
                    Temperature:     98.4°F
                    Pulse:           80 beats per minute
                    Respiration:     22/minute
                    Blood pressure:  130/84

**Laboratory and Diagnostic Tests:**
                    Red blood cell count:      3.9 million/µL
                    Hemoglobin:                11.0 g/dL
                    Hematocrit:                8.2%
                    Urine:                     negative
                    CAT scan:                  positive – degenerative disc disease
                    Approximate length of stay:  discharge third day

*continues*

Critical Pathway (continued)

## Nursing Diagnoses for Postoperative Days

| Day 1 | Day 2 | Day 3 |
|---|---|---|
| 1a. Risk for altered breathing pattern related to anesthesia. | 1a. Risk for altered breathing pattern related to immobility. | 1. Risk for ineffective airway clearance related to nonproductive cough. |
| 1b. Risk for ineffective airway clearance related to anesthesia, immobility, and ineffective coughing. | 1b. Risk for ineffective airway clearance related to ineffective cough and poor use of incentive inspirometer. | |
| 2a. Risk for fluid volume deficit related to wound dehiscence (bleeding). | 2a. Risk for fluid volume deficit related to wound dehiscence | 2a. Risk for fluid volume deficit related to wound dehiscence. |
| 2b. Risk for infection related to moisture and contamination of wound. | 2b. Risk for infection related to moisture and contamination of wound. | 2b. Risk for infection related to moisture and contamination of wound. |
| 3. Risk for sensory deficit related to nerve damage. | 3. Risk for sensory deficit related to nerve trauma. | 3a. Risk for sensory deficit related to nerve damage. |
| 4. Risk for altered elimination related to decrease muscle tone (detrusor muscle) from anesthesia and immobility. | 4. Risk for altered elimination related to decreased muscle tone (immobility). | 3b. Risk for activity intolerance related to nerve damage and fear. |
| 5. Risk for altered nutrition related to vomiting (anesthesia). | 5. Risk for acute pain (severe) related to ineffective use of PCA medication. | 4. Risk for knowledge deficit related to self-care management in hospital and at home. |
| 6. Risk for severe acute pain related to surgical intervention. Risk for activity intolerance related to sensory deficit, immobility, and fear. | 6. Risk for activity intolerance related to sensory deficit and fear. | |
| 7. Risk for knowledge deficit related to self-care management in hospital and at home. | 7. Risk for knowledge deficit related to self-care management in hospital and at home. | |

continues

| Post Op Day 1 | Y | N | Post Op Day 2 | Y | N | Post Op Day 3 | Y | N | Discharge Teaching | Y | N |
|---|---|---|---|---|---|---|---|---|---|---|---|
| 1a. Vital signs within normal range (assess q 15 minutes × 4 then q 1 hr × 4, if stable assess q 4 hrs) | | | 1a. Vital signs within normal range (assess every 4 hrs) | | | 1a. Vital signs normal (assess before discharge) | | | 1. Positive outcome of surgery reemphasized | | |
| 1b. Oxygen delivery patent (examine at least q 1 hr) | | | 1b. Oxygen 90 to 100 (oxygen discontinued) | | | 1b. Demonstrate proper use of incentive inspirometer increase fluids to 6 glasses a day. | | | 2. Importance in keeping incision dry to prevent infection discussed | | |
| 2. Dressing clean and dry (assess at least q 2 hrs) | | | 1c. Using inspirometer successfully (every 1 to 2 hrs) | | | 2. Dressing change (suture line approximated) | | | 3. Proper body mechanics discussed and demonstrated (avoid bending, stretching, lifting, stoop to pick up objects) | | |
| 3. Neurological findings within normal limits. (Perform neurological assessment q 15 minutes × 4 then q 1 hr × 4 if stable check every 4 hrs include capillary refill  sensation edema ability to move extremity) | | | 2. Dressing clean and dry (assess at least every 2 hrs) | | | 3. Neurological findings negative (able to walk with minimal to no assistance in hallway) | | | 4. Problems of overweight discussed (one problem, back pain including problems of the spine) | | |
| 4. Voided within 8 hours post op. (check for bladder distent on q 4 hrs to 6 hrs, and 8 hrs post op. If unable to void collaborate for catheterization) | | | 3. Neurological findings negative (assess at least every 4 hrs) | | | 4. Voiding spontaneously (output approximates intake) | | | 5. Importance of weight reduction discussed (avoid overeating, do not eat between meals, do not eat at night) | | |
| 5. Tolerating liquids/fluids when awake, oriented × 3 denies nausea (check gag reflex and complaints of nausea about 4 hrs post op) before feeding | | | 4. Voiding spontaneously intake approximate output (if Foley catheter in situ removed today) | | | 5. Taking extra fluids, eating regular diet (importance of eating balanced meal, and drinking 6 to 8 glasses of water explained) | | | 6. Drink 6 to 8 glasses of water daily, Discuss a plan of exercise with your doctor (information given) | | |

*continues*

Critical Pathway (continued)

## Goals/Interventions

## Discharge Teaching

| Post Op Day 1 | Y | N | Post Op Day 2 | Y | N | Post Op Day 3 | Y | N | Discharge Teaching | Y | N |
|---|---|---|---|---|---|---|---|---|---|---|---|
| 6. Using incentive inspirometer effectively at least q 1 to 2 hrs (teach effective use and rationale) | | | 5. Taking extra fluids— eating soft diet at least 50% (importance of not overeating explained) Hemoglobin 10.0 g/dL Hematocrit 37% | | | 6. Method of pain control reemphasized; self administration of medication explained | | | 7. Keep all scheduled appointments with your doctor | | |
| 7. Rates pain at 3 to 2 and tolerable (teach use of patient control anesthesia—PCA) | | | 6. Pain level 2 to 3 engaging in activities in daily living (discontinue PCA pump) Teach other methods of pain control; nonpharmacological/ pharmacological. | | | 7. Reemphasize reasons for anticoagulant and muscle relaxant | | | 8. Report all problems to your doctor immediately (temperature above 101° F, wetness or bleeding pain at operation site, other concerns) | | |
| 8. Able to stand at bedside with aid of physical therapist | | | 7. Explain reasons for all medications (anticoagulant, muscle relaxant and stool softener) | | | | | | | | |
| 9. Verbalizes satisfaction with outcome of operation (implement client teaching on satisfactory results of surgery) | | | | | | | | | | | |

## Revising the Nursing Care Plan after the Verbal Report

Review the following Nursing Care Plan for Mr. RB.

You prepared this care plan the evening before for your client (Mr. RB). The following day, you have your clinical experience from 0645 to 1430. You sequence your actions on your arrival to your unit as follows:

1. Listen to the morning report:

   Suppose the nurse states "Mr. RB, medical diagnosis: chronic obstructive pulmonary disease (COPD), Room 459, client had a good night's sleep. Vital signs were T 99° P 100 R 30, BP 140/90. Oxygen decreased to 2 liters per minute via nasal cannula."

2. Revision of the nursing care plan:

   You would now need to revise your care plan; you could not implement it as previously written because the client's condition has changed. The change in status would most likely be confirmed after you have done another assessment of your client.

3. Suppose the client states "I am breathing better."

   Short-term goal: Client will continue to demonstrate improved breathing, 20–26 respirations per minute. Color will be brighter pink.

   Long-term goal: Client's breathing will decrease to 18 to 20 breaths per minute. Review the original care plan for Mr. RB.

Now review the care plan for Mr. RB as revised following the morning report (see pp. 152–153).

**Client's Initial RB**  
**Room # 459**  
**Age 65**

## Nursing Care Plan

**Medical Diagnosis: Chronic Obstructive Pulmonary Disease (COPD)**

| Ordered & Selected Data | Nursing Diagnosis | Goals | Interventions | Rationale |
|---|---|---|---|---|
| Subjective: Client states "I can't breathe." | Altered breathing pattern related to altered lung ventilation and evidenced by restlessness & respirations of 45 beats per minute | Short term: Client will demonstrate improved breathing 28–30 respirations within 1 hour. Color will be less ashen (pale pink). | Independent Nursing Functions:<br>• Continue to nurse in high Fowler's position.<br>• Reassure client that everything is being done to improve condition:<br>—Stay with client.<br>—Adjust $O_2$ as needed.<br>—Apply cool cloth to forehead.<br>—Monitor VS q15 minutes<br>—Report condition as necessary. | Provides comfort<br><br>Facilitates breathing<br><br>Develops trust<br>Decreases anxiety<br><br><br>Decreases temperature<br>Provides for reassessment |
| Objective: Color ashen<br><br>T 100.2<br>P 110<br>R 45<br>BP 160/100<br><br>Lying in high Fowler's position—restless<br>$O_2$ via nasal cannula at 3 liters per minute | | Long term: Client's breathing will decrease to 20–25 beats per minute within 6 hours. | Dependent<br>Give medications as ordered.<br>Administer IV fluids as ordered.<br>Implement new orders.<br>Collaborative<br>Discuss $O_2$ therapy with therapist as necessary. | Medications & IV fluids are generally prescribed to improve the client's condition and prevent or improve dehydration.<br>Antibiotics treat infection or are given prophylactically. |
| Lung fields reveal: Crackles & rales in lower bases bilaterally<br>Hemoglobin—10 g/dL<br>Hematocrit—31% | Ineffective airway clearance related to nonproductive cough—tenacious sputum & generalized weakness & inability to cough effectively | Crackles & rhonchi will be less audible within 6 hours. | Independent<br>• Increase fluid intake:<br>800 cc 0700–1500<br>500 cc 1500–2300<br>200 cc 2300–0700<br>Encourage use of inspirometer q 1 to 2 hours if ordered.<br>Encourage coughing & deep breathing every 2 hours. | Loosens secretion from respiratory tract<br><br><br>Promotes alveolar gas exchange |

*Reference:* Phipps et al. (1999). *Medical-surgical nursing.*

**Client's Initial RB** **Age 65** **Nursing Care Plan (Revised after Verbal Report)**
**Room # 459** **Medical Diagnosis: Chronic Obstructive Pulmonary Disease (COPD)**

| Ordered & Selected Data | Nursing Diagnosis | Goals | Interventions | Rationale |
|---|---|---|---|---|
| Subjective: Client states "I am breathing better." <br><br> Objective: Color pale pink <br><br> T 99 <br> P 100 <br> R 30 <br> BP 140/90 <br><br> Lying in semi-Fowler's position—more relaxed <br> $O_2$ via nasal cannula at 2 liters per minute | Altered breathing pattern related to altered lung ventilation evidenced by respirations of 30 beats per minute | Short term: Client will continue to demonstrate improved breathing 20–26 respirations within 1 hour. Color will be brighter pink. <br><br> Long term: Client's breathing will decrease to 18–20 breaths per minute within 6 hours | Independent Nursing Functions: <br> • Continue to nurse in semi-Fowler's position: <br> • Reassure client that treatment regimen has begun to work and that his condition has shown improvement. <br> • Observe client's condition every 1–2 hours <br> • Adjust $O_2$ as needed. <br> • Apply cool cloth to forehead if needed. <br> • Monitor VS q2hours. <br> • Report condition as necessary. <br> Dependent <br> Give medications as ordered. <br> Administer IV fluids as ordered. <br> Implement new orders. <br> Collaborative <br> Discuss $O_2$ therapy with therapist as necessary. | Provides comfort <br><br> Facilitates breathing <br><br> Develops trust <br><br> Decreases anxiety <br><br> Decreases temperature <br><br> Provides for reassessment <br><br> Medications & IV fluids are generally prescribed to improve the client's condition and prevent or improve dehydration. |
| Lung fields reveal: Crackles & rales in lower bases bilaterally <br> Hemoglobin 10 g/dL <br> Hematocrit 31% | Ineffective airway clearance related to nonproductive cough—tenacious sputum & generalized weakness & inability to cough effectively | Crackles & rhonchi will be less audible within 6 hours | Independent <br> • Increase fluid intake: <br> 800 cc—0700–1500 <br> 500 cc—1500–2300 <br> 200 cc—2300–0700 <br> Encourage use of inspirometer (if ordered) q 1 to 2 hours (may collaborate if not ordered). <br> Encourage coughing & deep breathing every 2 hours. | Loosens secretion from respiratory tract <br><br> Promotes alveolar gas exchange |

*Reference:* Phipps et al. (1999). *Medical-surgical nursing.*

153

## KEY TERMS

**client's response**—The outcome of the nursing intervention (subjective and objective).

**client's status**—The present existing illness/wellness condition of the client.

**critical pathway**—Guideline that outlines specific expectations for a client's recovery on a day-by-day basis.

**existing need**—The client's present condition that warrants a specific nursing intervention.

**flow sheet**—Commercially prepared or institution designed forms that enable documentation of client outcomes with accuracy, efficiency, and in a timely manner.

**legal aspect**—That which may provide a source for litigation.

**rationale**—The scientific reason for performing a specific nursing intervention.

**recording**—Documentation that describes the results of the implementation. Recording may be done in any one of several charting formats. Health-care institutions specify the recording format to be used.

**underlying principle**—The reason for an action and the benefits to be derived by the client.

**verbal report**—Information shared about client's condition from one nurse to another, commonly at the change of shifts.

## NURSING CHECKLIST

### The Verbal Report
- Listen carefully to the change of shift report before implementing your previously written nursing interventions.
- Take notes as the nurse gives the report.
- Ask for clarification of information that was missed or unclear.
- Change your interventions to correspond to the new information that you receive.
- Review your revised nursing care plan with your instructor before implementation.

### The Rationale
- Always have a scientific base for each intervention.
- Always write the rationale beside each intervention. Use this information for teaching purposes. Remember to explain the procedure to the client and give the reason for the action.

### The Recording

- Always record/chart sequentially. Remember that information recorded as soon as possible after the activity is generally more accurate.
- Use the method of charting required by your unit.
- Become familiar and comfortable with all the charting methods discussed in this chapter. This will help you to work within given time constraints, be more accurate, and avoid undue frustration.

### Legal Concerns

- Remember that accurate, clear, and concise charting is less likely to lead to questions about professional behavior and competence.
- Remember to draw a straight line through an error, initial the error, and rewrite the correct information.
- Erasing is illegal and causes suspicion.

### The Flow Sheets

- Flow sheets are meant to save time and energy. Study them carefully and check all areas that pertain to your client. Be accurate and avoid duplication.

## CHAPTER SUMMARY

Implementation means to carry out the interventions that were written to meet the identified goals of a specific client. Implementation requires careful study and restudy. Nursing actions should be based on a nursing care plan revised according to the verbal report and the client's status (which should be ascertained through reassessment). A scientific rationale is required for every nursing action taken. For each action, client teaching should convey the reason before, during, and after the action. Accurate, clear, and precise documentation is required after every action and should follow the format required by the health-care institution. Flow sheets should be carefully studied and accurately completed to provide needed information and prevent duplication.

## REVIEW QUESTIONS

Choose the one best answer for each of the following questions.

1. Implementation is
   a. the evaluation phase of the nursing process.
   b. most closely related to DAR charting.

c. mostly connected to the subjective statements the client makes.

d. the action step in the nursing process.

2. Which of the following best describes the verbal report?

a. Questions the client asks about the treatment plan.

b. Idiosyncrasies voiced by the client.

c. Information about client status shared between nurses.

d. Identical information given to family members.

3. The rationale is best described as:

a. scientific reason for an action.

b. objective explanation of a phenomenon.

c. legal implications.

d. errors that are justifiable.

4. What client behaviors are likely to occur when they understand the underlying principles for a specific treatment regimen?

a. Trust

b. Withdrawal

c. Anger

d. Happiness

5. Proper documentation is most likely to prevent

a. inebriation.

b. duplication.

c. burnout.

d. anxiety.

6. Which of the following best describes the "S" in SOAP documentation?

a. Sublingual

b. Subtraction

c. Subjective

d. Silence

7. What is one benefit of narrative charting?

a. More comprehensive

b. Less comprehensive

c. Can all be done at the end of a shift

d. Always self-explanatory

8. Which method of charting most often needs to be supported by flow sheets?

   a. Computerized

   b. Narrative

   c. SOAPIER

   d. Focus

9. What action should the nurse take when an error is made in charting?

   a. Discard the previous record and recopy all entries.

   b. Draw a line through the incorrect portion, mark error, initial that section, and write the correct information.

   c. Draw two lines through the incorrect portion, sign your name, and write the correct information.

   d. Leave the charting with error uncorrected.

10. When is the best method of recording client information?

   a. At the end of a shift

   b. Sequentially

   c. As soon as possible

   d. Every 4 hours

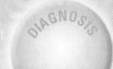

# Evaluation

## Objectives

Upon completion of this chapter, you should be able to:

- Utilize the steps of the evaluation phase.
- Differentiate between met and unmet outcome criteria/goals.
- Discuss rationale for exiting or retaining the client.
- Discuss the process of reassessment, rediagnosis, replanning, and putting the care plan together again.
- Discuss reevaluation.
- Describe the nursing process as a cycle.
- Identify ways of incorporating critical pathways into the nursing process.
- Discuss interdisciplinary care planning.

cycle                                    reassess
evaluation                               steps of the evaluation phase
outcome criteria

Your primary aim in writing the component parts of the care plan was to have positive outcomes for the client. You diligently assessed the client data, formulated a problem list (the nursing diagnoses), planned your goals/outcome criteria (those things you desired your client to achieve), planned your strategies, and implemented these strategies. Now you are at the end of the care plan—the **evaluation** phase. You are now to determine if the goals or **outcome criteria** are met and if the client's problems are solved and the extent to which they are met, whether totally or partially.

## DETERMINING THE RESULTS

The evaluation phase means that you must determine if the goals for the client are met. The **steps of the evaluation phase** require you to reexamine your:

- Assessment for relevance to the nursing diagnoses
- Nursing diagnoses for relevance to the goals and interventions
- Implementation for timing and completeness

Next, you are to look critically at the results (the outcome/goals). If the goals are met, you will detect positive changes in the client's physiologic condition and/or psychologic changes in the client's behavior.

See example care plan with goals met.

### Outcome Criteria (Goals) Met: Exiting the Client

When the goals are met, both client and nurse feel satisfaction. In discussing the completion of therapy with the client, you should allow time for the client to express his or her feelings about the care received. You will reaffirm positive comments and deal with any negative comments in a professional manner. Convey both your satisfaction and the health-care team's to the client. This is the time to discuss subsequent plans of care, such as discharge plans. Be sure both client and family members understand the discharge protocol, including (1) medications (name, dosage, times of administration, side effects,

| Ordered & Selected Data | Nursing Diagnosis | Goals | Interventions | Rationale | Evaluation |
|---|---|---|---|---|---|
| Subjective: Client states "I am breathing better." Objective: Color pale pink  T 99  P 100  R 30  BP 140/90  Lying in semi-Fowler's position—more relaxed  O₂ via nasal cannula at 2 liters per minute | Altered breathing pattern related to altered lung ventilation evidenced by respirations of 30 beats per minute | Short term: Client will continue to demonstrate improved breathing 20–26 respirations within 1 hour. Color will be brighter pink.  Long term: Client's breathing will decrease to 18–20 breaths per minute within 6 hours | Independent Nursing Functions: • Continue to nurse in semi-Fowler's position: • Reassure client that treatment regimen has begun to work and that his condition has shown improvement. ◦ Observe client condition every 1–2 hours ◦ Adjust O₂ as needed. ◦ Apply cool cloth to forehead if needed. ◦ Monitor VS q2hours. ◦ Report condition as necessary. Dependent Give medications as ordered. Administer IV fluids as ordered. Implement new orders. Collaborative Discuss O₂ therapy with therapist as necessary. | Provides comfort  Facilitates breathing  Develops trust  Decreases anxiety  Decreases temperature  Provides for reassessment  Medications & IV fluids are generally prescribed to improve the client's condition and prevent or improve dehydration. | Short term goal met: Client states "This cool cloth on my head really feels good; the oxygen is less troublesome than I thought." Temperature 99.0°F, pulse 100, respirations 26, color brighter pink. Voiced comfort in semi-Fowler's position.  Long term goals met: temperature 98.8°F, pulse 86, respirations 20, crackles and rales much less audible in both lower bases of the lungs. |
| Lung fields reveal: Crackles & rales in lower bases bilaterally  Hemoglobin 10 g/dL  Hematocrit 31% | Ineffective airway clearance related to nonproductive cough—tenacious sputum & generalized weakness & inability to cough effectively | Crackles & rhonchi will be less audible within 6 hours | Independent • Increase fluid intake: 800 cc—0700–1500 500 cc—1500–2300 200 cc—2300–0700 Encourage use of inspirometer q 1 to 2 hours. Encourage coughing & deep breathing every 2 hours. | Loosens secretion from respiratory tract  Promotes alveolar gas exchange | |

*Reference:* Phipps et al. (1999). *Medical-surgical nursing.*

and number of refills), (2) diet therapy (food and water with necessary restrictions), (3) other therapy and treatments such as physical therapy and dressing changes and exercise protocol, (4) time and date of return to the physician (including the physician's name, address, and telephone number), and (5) conditions to report to the physician prior to the appointment date, such as elevated temperature, increased pain, change in condition of wound, intolerance of medication, or any other concerns the client may have. You should write the discharge instructions on the discharge summary sheet. You will thoroughly discuss these instructions with the client and caregivers in a teaching session and have the client sign the form. Allow time for the client to read the form and ask questions. Give the client a legible copy of the form at the end of the teaching session. Escort the client with his or her belongings to the point of pick up according to agency protocol. This part of the evaluation process, which includes discharging the client, is called exiting the client or completing the plan of care.

## Outcome Criteria (Goals) Not Met: Retaining the Client

The process of determining if the goals/outcome criteria are not met is the same as identifying met goals. When the goals are not met, you need to **reassess** each step and critically ask:

- Was the correct data collected?
- Was the collected data complete?
- Was the collected data individualized?
- Were the right diagnoses made?
- Were the goals relevant and realistic?
- Were the right interventions selected?
- Was the implementation consistent with nursing standards?
- Were the interventions prioritized?
- Were the interventions timely and sequential?
- Were the interventions individualized?

During the reassessment phase, the nursing care plan continues to guide care for the client.

## Reassessment and Rediagnosis

Reassessment requires you to do the following:

- Critically look at the data for factual information.
- Collect additional data from charts, laboratory and diagnostic tests, family, client, and the health-care team.

- Reexamine the client by performing another physical assessment and another interview.
- Reassemble the new data and incorporate the old data as appropriate.
- Validate the new data.
- Arrange the data according to priority.
- Identify patterns.
- Formulate new diagnoses and examine both the old and the new for the PRS factors—the problem, related factors, and the signs and symptoms. For example: "altered breathing pattern related to hyperventilation evidenced by respirations of 40, dizziness, and tingling in fingers."
- Compare these nursing diagnoses with identifying characteristics. For your nursing diagnoses to be correct, the signs and symptoms you identified should correspond with at least three of the signs and symptoms listed in the defining chaacteristics.

## Replanning: Putting It All Together Again

You will need to reexamine your goals/outcome criteria to determine if they were:

- Relevant
- Realistic
- Client centered
- Within acceptable time constraints

You may need to write new goals. Be sure to address all requirements for proper goal writing. You should now rework the previous interventions and include any new ones you determine to be necessary. Use your critical thinking, problem-solving, and decision-making skills. Now you are ready to implement the new interventions. Be sure to deal with the most critical issues first. As you work with the client, encourage him or her to share information about feelings and concerns. Confirm positive and/or negative results. Work in an acceptable time frame and complete all tasks according to your plan (which should include all physicians' orders).

## Reevaluation

Examine the outcomes and determine if the new revised goals/outcome criteria are met. Remember that this examination begins during your implementation where you gain clues of positive and/or negative outcome achievements. This allows you to make adjustments as you progress. With a well-developed care plan you should achieve the desired outcomes—changes in the client's physical and emotional states leading to client and nursing satisfaction. You should now write "goals met" with some clarification of your observations that confirmed this conclusion. Next, follow the steps previously described for exiting the client from the process.

## THE NURSING PROCESS CYCLE

By this time you should be convinced that the nursing process is a **cycle** that requires correct fitting together of all the component parts. For the cycle to be complete and the outcome positive, you must work decisively and competently with each part. Continually compare each part of the cycle as you proceed to the end. If at the end you are not successful, you must begin all over again. Throughout the cycle there must be critical thinking, problem solving, and decision making. There must be client and nurse satisfaction before you stop the process and exit the client.

## INCORPORATING CRITICAL PATHWAYS INTO THE NURSING PROCESS

See example care plan in Chapter 5, page 147.
See revised care plan in Chapter 5, page 152.

## KEY TERMS

**cycle**—Each part impacts each other. If the data is incorrect, so will the diagnoses, goals, interventions, implementation, and subsequently, the outcome criteria (goal). Working the process/care plan in reverse, the sequencing should be clear. The result should be the same.

**evaluation**—Analyze the goal(s) (not the nursing interventions) to determine whether they are met or not met.

**outcome criteria**—Term used interchangeably with goal.

**reassess**—Look at all data sources and data collected as many times as you need to do this until the goal is realized—critically think.

**steps of the evaluation phase**—This is the last phase of the nursing process. Throughout the process, you critically look at all developments and refine the care plan to address changes. As the final step you analyze the entire process to determine if the goals are met.

# NURSING CHECKLIST

- Outcome criteria/goals are met.
  The desired outcome for the client is realized. This means there was direct correlation between the component parts of this nursing process (data, nursing diagnosis, planning [goals, interventions, and implementations]). In addition, critical thinking, problem solving, and decision making were decisively utilized. The client can now be discharged. Satisfaction should be felt both by client and health-care givers.
- Outcome criteria/goals are not met.
  Repeat the process using critical thinking, problem-solving, and decision-making skills to reassess each step to determine incongruencies in the cycle. The client is retained and the refining process is continued until the expected outcome is realized–goal met.
- Reassessment
  When the goal is not met, you may need to review the client's record again, talk to significant others and the client to confirm or revise prerecorded statements, and/or do another physical assessment. After this is accomplished, you revise the nursing diagnoses and planning (goals and interventions), and determine measures for implementation. The correct scientific rationale for each intervention will help you focus your activities and realize the goals.
- Reevaluation
  Subsequent evaluations are done every time the plan has to be reworked.
- The nursing process cycle
  The component parts must correlate (relate to each other). Use a ruler to draw a line from data to evaluation. Work forward from data to evaluation and again from the evaluation column to the data column. There should be correct sequencing of the parts.
- Critical pathways
  All plans of care are developed by interdisciplinary teams. They identify specific time frames to show where the client should be on a health/illness continuum on a given day or given week. They are used for clients who can be expected to show progressive recovery and generally not for clients with debilitating illnesses. The critical pathway plans should guide your critical thinking as you draw conclusions about goals that are realized as opposed to goals that are not. You should also be able to format a nursing process care plan from one that is developed according to critical pathways.

## CHAPTER SUMMARY

The evaluation phase reveals the true cyclical nature of the nursing process. It is in this phase that you determine if the data was truly representative of the diagnoses and vice versa. It causes you to reexamine the planning phase for:

1. Goals for relevancy, individualization, time constraints, long and short term, and measurability.
2. Interventions that focused on actions to meet each goal. The evaluation phase forces you to look at the way you implemented your interventions (nursing actions).

Finally, it causes you to decide if your goals were met and the benefits and satisfaction to the client and the satisfaction to the nurse.

The evaluation phase has another impact. It helps you decide on how to rework the cycle from data collection through evaluation if the goals were not met (retain the client) and how to exit (discharge the client) if the goals are met.

## REVIEW QUESTIONS

1. Which of the following best describes the evaluation phase?
   a. Critical thinking sequentially from data through planning, intervention, implementation, and evaluation.
   b. Critical thinking through planning, intervention, implementation, and evaluation.
   c. Goals met.
   d. Goals not met.

2. Which of the following describes a met goal?
   a. Client voices satisfaction with the nurses' performance.
   b. The client voiced relief of the pain within 1 hour of the pain medication and ambulated with his or her walker without complaint.
   c. The client asked to see his doctor, stating "I am ready to be discharged."
   d. Client performed his own bath.

3. An unmet goal can best be described as which of the following?
   a. No visible change in the client's condition (problem).
   b. Client states "I feel fine."

c. Client developed a temperature of 101°F.

d. Client's urine was amber.

4. What is the course of action when a goal is met?

a. Share the satisfaction of the health-care team with the client and complete the discharge plan.

b. Counsel the client about unhealthful practices and challenge him or her never to resume previous practices. Complete the discharge plan.

c. Counsel the client of his or her responsibility to society and his or her responsibility to be a good role model.

d. Compliment the client for the quick recovery, discuss the impact of his or her illness on the state treasury and complete the discharge planning.

5. What is your understanding of the best time for exiting the client from the treatment plan?

a. Partial recovery.

b. Goal not met.

c. Client's discharge request.

d. Goal met.

6. What is your understanding of putting the care plan together again?

a. All goals are met. Reworking the care plan from data collection through assessment.

b. The evaluation phase is complete.

c. Goals are not met. Rework the care plan from data through evaluation.

d. Implementation is incomplete.

7. What should the nurse be looking for during reassessment?

a. Complete, relevant, and reliable data.

b. Any evidence of criminal record.

c. Any evidence of sibling rivalry.

d. Ability to run the marathon.

8. During replanning, examination should be determined whether goals are

a. too long.

b. current.

c. individualized.

d. met.

9. What is your understanding of reevaluation?

   a. Rework all component parts of the nursing process.
   b. Rework the goals.
   c. Examine the client's concerns.
   d. Reexamine the data.

10. Key terms are best described as

   a. words that are difficult to understand.
   b. terms that will provide clear understanding within the context of a statement.
   c. terms that were never used before.
   d. sentences peculiar to a certain client.

# Appendix NANDA Nursing Diagnoses 2001–2002

Activity intolerance

Activity intolerance, Risk for

Adjustment, Impaired

Airway clearance, Ineffective

Allergy response, Risk for latex

Anxiety

Anxiety, Death

Aspiration, Risk for

Body image, Disturbed

Body temperature, Risk for imbalanced

Bowel incontinence

Breastfeeding, Effective

Breastfeeding, Ineffective

Breastfeeding, Interrupted

Breathing pattern, Ineffective

Cardiac output, Decreased

Caregiver role strain

Caregiver role strain, Risk for

Communication, Impaired verbal

Confusion, Acute

Confusion, Chronic

Constipation

Constipation, Perceived

Constipation, Risk for

Coping, Community, Ineffective

Coping, Community, Readiness for enhanced

Coping, Defensive

Coping, Family, Compromised

Coping, Family, Disabled

Coping, Family, Readiness for enhanced

Coping, Ineffective

Conflict, Decisional (specify)

Conflict, Parental role

Denial, Ineffective

Dentition, Impaired

Development, Risk for delayed

Diarrhea

Disuse syndrome, Risk for

Diversional activity, Deficient

Dysreflexia, Autonomic

Energy field, Disturbed

Environmental interpretation syndrome, Impaired

Failure to thrive, Adult

Falls, Risk for

Family processes, Dysfunctional: Alcoholism

Family processes, Interrupted

Fatigue

Fear

Fluid volume, Deficient

Fluid volume, Excess

Fluid volume, Risk for deficient

Fluid volume, Risk for imbalanced

Gas exchange, Impaired

Grieving, Anticipatory

Grieving, Dysfunctional

Growth and development, Delayed

Growth, Risk for disproportionate

Health Maintenance, Ineffective

Health-seeking behaviors (specify)

Home maintenance, Impaired

Hopelessness

Hyperthermia

Hypothermia

Identity, Disturbed personal

Incontinence, Functional urinary

Incontinence, Reflex urinary

Incontinence, Stress urinary

Incontinence, Total urinary

Incontinence, Urge urinary

Incontinence, Urge urinary, Risk for

Infant behavior, Disorganized

Infant behavior, Readiness for enhanced organized

Infant behavior, Risk for disorganized

Infant feeding pattern, Ineffective

Infection, Risk for

Injury, Perioperative positioning, Risk for

Injury, Risk for

Intracranial adaptive capacity, Decreased

Knowledge, Deficient

Loneliness, Risk for

Memory, Impaired

Mobility, Impaired bed

Mobility, Impaired physical

Mobility, Impaired wheelchair

Nausea

Noncompliance (specify)

Nutrition, Imbalanced: Less than body requirements

Nutrition, Imbalanced: More than body requirements

Nutrition, Imbalance: More than body requirements, Risk for

Oral mucous membrane, Impaired

Pain, Acute

Pain, Chronic

Parent/infant/child attachment, Risk for impaired

Parenting, Impaired

Parenting, Impaired, Risk for

Peripheral neurovascular dysfunction, Risk for

Poisoning, Risk for

Post-trauma syndrome

Post-trauma syndrome, Risk for

Powerlessness

Powerlessness, Risk for

Protection, Ineffective

Rape-trauma syndrome

Rape-trauma syndrome, Compound reaction

Rape-trauma syndrome, Silent reaction

Relocation stress syndrome

Relocation stress syndrome, Risk for

Role performance, Ineffective

Self-care deficit, Bathing/hygiene

Self-care deficit, Dressing/grooming

Self-care deficit, Feeding

Self-care deficit, Toileting

Self-esteem, Low, Chronic

Self-esteem, Low, Situational

Self-esteem, Low, Situational, Risk for

Self-mutilation

Self-mutilation, Risk for

Sensory perception, Disturbed (specify)
   (Visual, auditory, kinesthetic, gustatory, tactile,
   olfactory)

Sexual dysfunction

Sexuality patterns, Ineffective

Skin integrity, Impaired

Skin integrity, Impaired, Risk for

Sleep deprivation

Sleep pattern, Disturbed

Social interaction, Impaired

Social isolation

Sorrow, Chronic

Spiritual distress

Spiritual distress, Risk for

Spiritual well-being, Readiness for enhanced

Suffocation, Risk for

Suicide, Risk for

Surgical recovery, Delayed

Swallowing, Impaired

Therapeutic regimen management, Effective

Therapeutic regimen management, Ineffective

Therapeutic regimen management, Ineffective community

Therapeutic regimen management, Ineffective family

Thermoregulation, Ineffective

Thought process, Disturbed

Tissue integrity, Impaired

Tissue perfusion, Ineffective (specify type)

      (Renal, cerebral, cardiopulmonary, gastrointestinal, peripheral)

Transfer ability, Impaired

Trauma, Risk for

Neglect, unilateral

Urinary elimination, Impaired

Urinary retention

Ventilation, Impaired spontaneous

Ventilatory weaning response, Dysfunctional

Violence, Risk for other-directed

Violence, Risk for self-directed

Walking, Impaired

Wandering

Source: North American Nursing Diagnosis Association (2001). *Nursing diagnoses: Definitions and classifications, 2001–2002*. Philadelphia, PA: Author.

# Glossary

**actual nursing diagnosis**—A nursing diagnosis that displays specific signs and symptoms that relate to the client's problem.

**analyze**—To critically look at the component parts of the client data, determine their interrelatedness and their significance to the client's problems; to look critically at the selected data and the signs and symptoms it reveals and to determine the specific relationship to a particular NANDA diagnosis.

**assessment**—The beginning phase in the nursing process where patient data is collected. This forms the basis for the nursing diagnosis; relates to the data that you gather through the interview and the physical examination. It includes critical thinking, problem solving, and decision making in order to extrapolate that which is significant and reliable from that which is insignificant and unreliable.

**assessment tools**—Specific written guidelines (checklists) that guide the nurse in the comprehensive data collection from each client.

**baseline data**—Initial information gleaned from the client at the time of admission that facilitates the formulation of the medical diagnosis and the nursing diagnosis and confirms the need for further investigation such as laboratory and diagnostic tests and consultation from other experts.

**caring**—An inner feeling of wanting to do, wanting to help. It is identifying with all the client's concerns.

**client's response**—The outcome of the nursing intervention (subjective and objective).

**client's status**—The present existing illness/wellness condition of the client.

**closed questions**—Questions posed by nurse to the client that generate yes and no answers. Should be used only for that intent.

**collaborative problem**—The nursing diagnosis that may develop and will require teamwork in order to arrive at client solutions. The treatment plan is not solely in the nurse's realm of practice, but the nurse carries out nursing interventions in collaboration with physicians and other health-care providers such as the dietician, social worker, occupational therapist, and physical therapist. Collaborative problems are written preceded with the letters "PC," for example, "PC pneumonia" meaning "potential for complication."

**critical pathway**—Guideline that outlines specific expectations for a client's recovery on a day-by-day basis.

**critical thinking**–Is an active thought process that analyzes all parts of a problem, arrives at specific goals to be realized, makes decisions about appropriate interventions, and examines outcomes.

**cultural/spiritual**–Meeting specific needs of individual–holistic care.

**cycle**–Each part impacts each other. If the data is incorrect, so will the diagnoses, goals, interventions, implementation, and subsequently, the outcome criteria (goal). Working the process/care plan in reverse, the sequencing should be clear. The result should be the same.

**defining characteristics**–These are actual signs and symptoms that are manifested when a client has a specific problem or disease. They are scientifically proven; hence, they are used to categorize specific problems and disease processes. Nurses use them to verify selected nursing diagnoses.

**dependent nursing functions**–Nursing interventions carried out in response to a physician's orders.

**diagnosis**–The second phase of the nursing process in which the problems identified in the assessment are categorized from the NANDA approved list and named as present (actual) or likely to happen in a given situation (risk for).

**discharge goals**–Comprehensive benefits the client should derive while under your care and in the home setting.

**empathic listening**–Attentive listening. A posture maintained by the nurse throughout all client communication that makes the nurse cognizant of all that the client says. Empathic listening is verifiable by the nurse's restatement, confrontation, leading questions, and appropriate silence.

**empathy**–In-depth understanding of a person's feelings and concerns and the ability to share warmth and understanding through verbal and nonverbal communication (giving of self).

**etiology**–The factor that points out the cause for the problem/diagnosis.

**evaluation**–Examination that occurs throughout the nursing process to determine reliability of data, correctness of the nursing diagnosis, attainable goals, appropriate nursing interventions, and the realization of the expectations; analyze the goal(s) (not the nursing interventions) to determine whether they are met or not met.

**existing need**–The client's present condition that warrants a specific nursing intervention.

**flow sheet**–Commercially prepared or institution designed forms that enable documentation of client outcomes with accuracy, efficiency, and in a timely manner.

**focus**–The elimination of extraneous data and the pinpointing of the major factors that are causing the client's problem.

**goal**–A desired outcome.

**goals**–The benefit(s) the client should experience after the nursing intervention.

**implementation**–The carrying out of the listed interventions (performing the required nursing care) in order to realize the identified client goals.

**independent nursing functions**–The nursing interventions that are nurse specific. They do not necessarily need a physician's order. Most of them are scientifically proven to be effective when used to solve specific client care problems/diagnoses. They can be found in nursing textbooks.

**interpersonal**–Relationship between people. Ways in which people interact with one another that may be positive or negative.

**interrelatedness**–The relationship between parts. Determining how each part affects the other.

**intervention**–Actions that are taken to treat or solve a problem.

**interview**–A one-to-one relationship between the client and the nurse during which time information is collected and used to guide the physical assessment.

**intrapersonal**–Looking into one's self to determine feelings and attitudes about others.

**intuition**–Quick and ready insight that, in some situations, might give one a feeling of impending danger.

**legal aspect**–That which may provide a source for litigation.

**legal/ethical considerations**–Goals that focus on awareness of client's rights, privileges, and safety.

**long-term goals**–More than can be expected on the first day, but while the client is still in your care. May be written in collaboration with staff–if so, specify.

**need**–A desire within an individual that, if left unfulfilled, can cause anxiety and stress.

**nursing process**–A systematic way of assessing, planning, diagnosing, and evaluating patient care situations.

**open-ended questions**–Broad statements that encourage the client to explore and verbalize all feelings and concerns. These statements discourage yes and no answers.

**ordering and selecting/clustering**–Categorizing sections of client's data that correlate with one another. It includes what the client says during the interview (subjective data) and the signs that are found during the physical assessment (objective data). Both the subjective data and the objective data are ordered/clustered and used to determine the nursing diagnosis.

**outcome criteria**–Used interchangeably with goals; that which is expected during and at the end of the planned therapy.

**planning**–The phase of the nursing process where the assessment data and the nursing diagnosis are utilized in the formulation of client-centered goals and interventions in order to meet the client's needs. The health-care team and the client are actively involved in formulating the plan of care.

**possible nursing diagnosis**–Is written in a situation where the evidence for that problem did not exist prior to the client's accessing health care. However, because of the medical diagnosis, the possible problem/nursing diagnosis may develop.

**primary information**–Initial data collected from the client or significant others and verified by the physical assessment that leads to beginning nursing diagnosis or diagnoses and subsequently facilitates collaboration among the health care team.

**prioritizing**–Sequencing according to importance. Arranging according to urgency. Determining client's problems that require immediate action. Organizing problems and concerns on a continuum according to the immediacy of the need for intervention.

**priority/prioritize**–The clustering of patient data from most crucial (needs immediate attention) to least crucial (can be dealt with after the crucial problems are addressed). Goals are written to correspond with the nursing diagnoses prioritized list.

**problem**–Another name for the nursing diagnosis. The terms may be used together; for example, nursing diagnosis (problem).

**rationale**–The scientific reason for performing a specific nursing intervention.

**reassess**–Look at all data sources and data collected as many times as you need to do this until the goal is realized–critically think.

**recording**–The written account of the plan of care, individualized according to each client's need. Documentation that describes the results of the implementation. Recording may be done in any one of several charting formats. Health-care institutions specify the recording format to be used.

**risk nursing diagnosis**–Problems that a client might encounter because of diagnostic tests or other compromising situations of which the client may be subjected during the course of treatment, such as surgical interventions.

**sequencing**–All parts of the nursing process relate to each other–data, nursing diagnosis, goal, interventions, rationale evaluation (outcome criteria/ goal).

**short-term goals**–Those that can be expected during your interaction with the client on the first day.

**significant others**–Individuals within the client's circle of family members, friends, or associates who have knowledge about past and/or current behaviors and are willing to share information or give other assistance during the client's illness.

**standards of care**–Nursing care provided according to professional nursing standards designated by the American Nursing Association.

**steps of the evaluation phase**–This is the last phase of the nursing process. Throughout the process, you critically look at all developments and refine the care plan to address changes. As the final step you analyze the entire process to determine if the goals are met.

**syndrome diagnosis**–The term is used when the client has a chronic illness or suffers severe psychological trauma, either or both conditions may put the client at risk for many nursing diagnosis. These are written "at risk for."

**teaching goals**–Those goals that relate to the nursing diagnosis "knowledge deficit."

**underlying principle**–The reason for an action and the benefits to be derived by the client.

**valid data**–Client information, which is substantiated by the client or significant other's verbal communication and the physical assessment.

**verbal report**–Information shared about client's condition from one nurse to another, commonly at the change of shifts.

**wellness diagnosis**–A diagnosis written when the client is not then complaining of symptoms of a disease and related signs are not evident. The objective is to assist the client to maintain or reach even a higher state of health or performance.

# Bibliography

Alfaro-LeFevre, R. (1998). *Applying nursing process: A step-by-step guide*. Philadelphia: Lippincott.

Allan C.V. (1997). *Nursing process in collaborative practice: A problem solving approach*. Stamford, CT: Appleton & Lange.

Altman, G., Buchsel, P., & Coxon, V. (2000). *Fundamental and advanced nursing skills*. Clifton Park, NY: Delmar Learning.

American Nurses Association (1980). *Nursing and social policy statement*. Kansas City, MO: Author.

American Nurses Association (1991). *Standards of clinical nursing practice*. Kansas City, MO: Author.

American Nurses Association (1973). *Standards of nursing practice*. Kansas City, MO: Author.

Barnum, B., (1996). *Spirituality in nursing from traditional to new age*. New York: Springer.

Bates, B. (2002). *A guide to physical examination and history taking*. Philadelphia: Lippincott.

Beyea, S. (1996). *Critical pathways for collaborative nursing care*. Menlo Park, CA: Addison-Wesley.

Carpenito, L.J. (1997). *Handbook of nursing diagnosis*. Philadelphia: Lippincott.

Carpenito, L.J. (1995). *Nursing care plans and documentation: Nursing diagnoses and collaborative problems*. Philadelphia: Lippincott.

Carpenito, L.J. (2000). *Nursing diagnosis: Application to clinical practice*. Philadelphia: Lippincott.

Craven, R. & Hirnle, C. (2002). *Fundamentals of nursing: Human health and function*. Philadelphia: Lippincott.

Daniels, R. (2002). *Delmar's guide to laboratory and diagnostic tests*. Clifton Park, NY: Delmar Learning.

Doenges, M., Moorhouse, M., & Geissler-Murr, A. (2002). *Nursing care plans: Guidelines for individualizing patient care* (6th ed.). Philadelphia: F.A. Davis.

Doheny, M., Cook, C., & Stopper, M. (1992). *The Discipline of nursing: An introduction* (5th ed.). Norwalk, CT: Appleton & Lange.

Estes, M. (1998). *Health assessment and physical examination*. Clifton Park, NY: Delmar Learning.

Fitzgerald, M. (1994). *Nursing health assessment: Concepts and activities*. Springhouse, PA: Springhouse.

Fry, S., & Veatch, R. (2000). *Case studies in nursing ethics*. Boston: Jones and Bartlett.

Gaut, D.A., & Leininger, M.M. (1991). *Caring–The compassionate healer*. New York: National League for Nursing Press.

Gordon, M. (1998). *Manual of nursing diagnosis: Featuring Gordon's functional health patterns*. St. Louis, MO: C.V. Mosby.

Hall, J. (1996). *Nursing ethics and law*. Philadelphia: W.B. Saunders.

Husted, G., & Husted, J. (2001). *Ethical decision making in nursing and health care: The symphonological approach*. New York: Spring Publishing.

Iyer, P., Taptich, B., & Bernocchi-Losey, D. (1994). *Nursing process and nursing diagnosis*. Philadelphia: W.B. Saunders.

Kozier, B., Erb, G., Berman, A., & Burke, K. (2000). *Fundamentals of nursing: Concepts, process, and practice*. Upper Saddle River, NJ: Prentice Hall Health.

Lederer, J., Gail, L., & Moenik, B. (1993). *Care planning pocket guide: A nursing diagnosis approach*. Redwood, City CA: Addison Wesley Nursing.

Leininger, M.M. (1995). *Transcultural nursing: Concepts, theories, research and practices*. New York: McGraw-Hill.

Lewis, S., Heitkemper, M., & Dirksen, S. (2000). *Medical-surgical nursing: Assessment and management of clinical problems*. St. Louis, MO: C.V. Mosby.

Lindberg, J.B., Hunter, M.L., & Kruszewski, Ann Z. (1994). *Introductino to nursing: Concepts, issues, and opportunities*. Philadelphia: Lippincott.

McSherry, W. (2000). *Making sense of spirituality in nursing practice, An interactive approach*. Philadelphia: Churchill Livingston.

Miller, M.A. & Babcock, D.E. (1996). *Critical thinking applied to nursing*. St. Louis, MO: C.V. Mosby.

O'Brien, M.E. (1999). *Spirituality in nursing: Standing on holy ground*. Boston: Jones & Bartlett.

Phipps, W., Long, B., & Woods, N. (1999). *Medical-surgical nursing: Concepts and clinical practice*. St. Louis, Mo.: C.V. Mosby.

Potter, P., & Perry, A. (2002). *Fundamentals of nursing*. St. Louis, MO: C.V. Mosby.

Rubenfeld, M.G. & Scheffer, B.K. (1995). *Critical thinking in nursing: An interactive approach*. Philadelphia: Lippincott.

Smith, S., Duell, D., & Martin, C. (2000). *Clinical nursing skills: Basic to advanced skills*. Stamford, CT: Appleton & Lange.

Sorensen, K. & Luckman, J. (2001). *Basic nursing: A psychophysiologic approach*. Philadelphia: W.B. Saunders.

Taylor, E. (2002). *Spiritual care: Nursing theory, research, and practice*. Upper Saddle River, NJ: Prentice Hall.

Watson, J. (1994). *Applying the art and science of human caring*. New York: National League for Nursing.

Watson, J. (2002). *Assessing and measuring caring in nursing and health science*. New York: Springer.

Watson, J. & Ray, M.A. (1998). *The ethics of care and the ethics of cure: Synthesis in chronicity*. NewYork: National League for Nursing.

Wilkinson, J. (2000). *Nursing process and critical thinking*. Menlo Park, CA: Addison-Wesley Nursing.

# Index

An "f" following a page number indicates a figure. A "t" indicates a table.